CO-AOF-639

Responding to

AIDS

PSYCHOSOCIAL INITIATIVES

PROPERTY OF THE
CLINICAL SOCIAL
WORK INSTITUTE

Responding to
AIDS

PSYCHOSOCIAL INITIATIVES

Carl G. Leukefeld
and
Manuel Fimbres,
Editors

National Association of Social Workers, Inc.
Silver Spring, MD 20910
Dorothy V. Harris, *President* • Mark G. Battle, *Executive Director*

RC
607
.A26
R47
1987

Copyright © 1987 by the National Association of Social Workers, Inc.

All rights reserved. No part of this book may be reproduced or transmitted in any form or by any means, electronic or mechanical, including photocopying, recording, or by any information storage and retrieval system, without permission in writing from the publisher.

Library of Congress Cataloging-in-Publication Data

Responding to AIDS: psychosocial initiatives

  Includes bibliographies.
    1. AIDS (Disease)—Social aspects. 2. Social service.
I. Leukefeld, Carl G. II. Fimbres, Manuel.
III. National Association of Social Workers.
RC607.A26R47 1987   362.1'969792   87-15211
ISBN 0-87101-148-4

Printed in U.S.A.

Design by Dan Hildt, Graphics in General, Washington, D.C.

CONTENTS

RC
607
.A26
R47
1987

Preface

The psychosocial consequences of AIDS, the stigma placed on the two groups at highest risk of contracting AIDS (homosexuals and intravenous drug abusers), and the needs for education about and prevention of the disease have challenged social workers. Social work services to persons with AIDS and AIDS-related complex (ARC), to those infected with the human immunodeficiency virus (HIV), and to their families, friends, lovers, caretakers, and co-workers need to be developed and provided in collaboration with other health care professionals. Social workers can take leadership by exercising the competence and compassion of their profession.

Psychosocial co-factors may combine with the HIV infection to trigger and exacerbate the course of AIDS. Social work services must focus on those with HIV infection who are asymptomatic to help keep the disease from being triggered, on those with ARC to help inhibit a stress-related triggering of AIDS or to retard the development of AIDS, and on those with AIDS to help in the most humane way, especially in relation to death and dying.

The first and sometimes only sign that a person has AIDS may be a neuropsychiatric problem. Central nervous system dysfunctions associated with AIDS may result from direct infection with the virus. Symptoms ranging from memory loss to dementia are common. Social workers need to understand the impact of the virus on the central nervous system and work with all those who are involved with the person with AIDS.

Finally, social work services must be provided to those who voluntarily or involuntarily take the HIV-antibody test or are considering whether to take it, and to those who have taken the test and need to understand the ramifications of either a positive or negative result.

The projections for the future number of persons in this country who will contract AIDS, ARC, or seropositivity are ominous. Social workers can effectively address this devastating epidemic now and in the future. Until such time as there is a vaccine or cure, only education and prevention can reduce the numbers. Social workers must encourage changes in behavior, and maintenance of these changes over time, to reduce risk.

Because of the seriousness of the crisis and the response to it by the social work profession, the National Institute of Mental Health assisted the

National Association of Social Workers in the preparation of this publication. It is hoped that social workers will become knowledgeable about AIDS and will not only provide effective social work services to persons with AIDS-spectrum disorders but will give accurate information to others about AIDS, it transmission, and the implications of high-risk behavior in order to promote the prevention of AIDS.

JUAN R. RAMOS
National Institute of Mental Health
Rockville, Maryland

March 1987

Introduction

The AIDS epidemic poses tremendous challenges to health, mental health, and social work professionals as they work to identify and meet the complicated medical and psychosocial needs of persons with AIDS. Public health authorities have identified AIDS as today's major public health problem. At the Coolfont conference, conducted by the U.S. Public Health Service in June 1986, it was estimated that, by 1991, $8–$16 billion will be spent for the treatment of persons with AIDS and that, by the end of 1991, more than 270,000 persons will have contracted AIDS and 54,000 persons will be dying of it each year.

The AIDS challenge for social workers is obvious. Clearly, the lack of pharmacological, immunological, and medical interventions emphasizes the need for psychosocial and behavioral interventions—the traditional focus of social workers. At points during the life cycle of the disease, persons with AIDS are overwhelmed with stressful life events and fears for which they and their loved ones require specific information and help with developing strategies to cope and to reduce the stress they are experiencing. Thus, the challenge for social workers, like that for other helping professionals, is to provide services in an accepting, responsive, and nonthreatening manner.

Policies for Social Workers

The 1984 NASW Delegate Assembly adopted a policy statement on AIDS reaffirming that AIDS is a public health crisis and that social workers can help alleviate the crisis by pursuing actions in six areas:

■ Basic epidemiological and clinical research on AIDS.

■ The distribution of accurate information on treatment and the medical, financial, and psychosocial resources that are available.

■ The provision of comprehensive psychological and social supports to help persons with AIDS, their families, children, spouses, and loved ones.

■ The development of a comprehensive service delivery system to respond to the AIDS crisis, including suitable housing, home health care, and transportation services.

■ The protection of the civil rights and right to confidentiality of persons who are diagnosed as having AIDS or AIDS-related complex (ARC).

■ The protection by the helping professionals and appropriate licensing authorities of the eligibility for and receipt of benefits by persons with AIDS.

In July 1986, the AIDS Task Force of the New York City Chapter of NASW adopted the following guidelines for the ethical delivery of services to persons with AIDS to complement NASW's Policy Statment on AIDS:

1. All persons with AIDS, ARC, or a positive antibody test finding or for whom there is an unsubstantiated presumption that they have or have acquired AIDS shall have access to services offered by professional social workers.

2. Social workers in all practice settings and different levels of authority are obligated to become knowledgeable about the basic modes of transmission of the human immunodeficiency virus (HIV) and be prepared to educate and counsel peers, other professionals, and clients.

3. Consequently, all social workers should participate in periodic and continuous education and updating of their scientific knowledge about AIDS. They should also be familiar with effective ways to serve persons with AIDS and their family members, life partners, friends, and others.

4. Social workers should encourage and support the development by agencies of up-to-date written guidelines and procedures for their practice with people in the categories listed in item 1; such written statements should reflect the spirit of all items in these guidelines.

5. All social workers must respect the confidentiality of all written and oral communications between them and others who face AIDS, ARC, and related conditions. Special attention must be given to the protection of the anonymity of persons who take HIV antibody screening tests.

6. Social workers should particularly be concerned about the emotional impact and possible consequences to the human rights of people taking the HIV antibody test. They should make certain that the limits of the predictive value of such tests are known in advance by clients. Appropriate counseling should be offered to clients by social workers and other skilled professionals.

7. Social workers are obligated to report any breaches of confidentiality and anonymity with respect to clients in regard to any aspect of the testing or diagnosis of AIDS and ARC to the appropriate body of accountability specific in agency-written guidelines.

8. All social workers should become knowledgeable about the particular needs of people in the categories listed in item 1 for health and long-term care, income maintenance, preventive education programs, mental health services, legal assistance, housing, hospices, child care, schooling, recreation, and participation in and access to community services.

9. Social workers who can fulfill their job responsibilities should not be denied employment if they have AIDS or ARC, have tested positive on the antibody test, or are presumed to be in an at-risk group.

10. The highly stressful nature of social work practice with AIDS requires that social workers have appropriate supportive supervision, consultation with peers, and respite from the strain of work.

In addition, NASW's Commission on Education endorsed the policies on AIDS in the schools, adopted by the National Education Association (NEA) in October 1983, with three additions. (The NEA guidelines are consistent with those of the Centers for Disease Control, which call for a case-by-case assessment and review of students and school employees with AIDS.) NASW's additions to the NEA policy are that (1) social workers should be included in the assessment and review process, (2) in-service training about AIDS should be provided to school social workers and other pupil services personnel, and (3) particular attention should be given to the needs of children with AIDS who are too young to attend school or are special education students.

The Institute

This volume includes papers presented at an institute, hosted by the NASW Commission on Health and Mental Health and the National Committee on Lesbian and Gay Issues, on September 11, 1986, at the NASW National Conference on Clinical Social Work in San Francisco, California. The institute's title—"Responding to the Challenge of AIDS: Psychosocial Initiatives"—provides the flavor for this collection of papers, which were commissioned by NASW with sponsorship from the National Institute of Mental Health.

The three overall objectives of the institute and this volume are:

■ To identify what is known about the psychosocial issues accompanying AIDS and ARC through a review of the literature on practice and research in this area and an examination of psychosocial interventions.

■ To discuss professional roles required to meet the psychosocial needs of individuals, families, and communities and the training requirements to fill these roles.

■ To identify which services are needed and how they should be delivered, as well as the implications for developing social policies.

The Chapters

Ryan discusses the challenge of AIDS and the charge to the profession and to social work practitioners. Leukefeld and Battjes present an overview of the incidence and prevalence data on AIDS from the Centers for Disease Control and the projections for a vast increase inthe incidence and prevalence of AIDS by 1991. Schwartz reviews research on the psychosocial aspects of AIDS in two general categories: onset studies, which examine the impact of psychological experiences on health, and psychological needs studies, which explore the changed psychological and social situations of persons who have contracted AIDS or ARC. After describing the joint AIDS program of San Francisco General Hospital and the University of California at San Francisco and presenting the program's demographic data, Macks discusses the psychosocial needs of persons with AIDS and the range of services to meet these needs. She also clarifies the implications of these needs for the delivery of services to persons with AIDS and advocates public policies to address the AIDS epidemic. Newmark and Taylor draw on their clinical experience as evidence that practitioners must apply new concepts of the family in working with persons with AIDS. In addition, they review clinical issues and interweave their discussion of interventions with case-management tasks and case examples.

Chachkes describes the devastating nature of AIDS by describing the effects of the disease on women and children and presenting two case illustrations involving a child with AIDS and children of parents with AIDS. Furthermore, she identifies the role of social workers as providers of assistance with housing, income maintenance, medical care, home care, long-term care, foster care, legal services, and counseling, as well as mental health services.

Jue focuses her presentation on three minority groups—Asians, blacks, and Hispanics—which make up over 28 percent of the U.S. population and approximately 40 percent of persons with AIDS. She discusses the sociocultural issues involved in working with minority persons with AIDS, the specific service and counseling needs of these groups, and the obstacles to treatment. Moynihan and Christ present social and psychological barriers to the treatment of people with AIDS and problems that are emerging from the research treatment of AIDS. They present the development of professional and other liaisons as a framework for the provision of comprehensive interventions.

Guidelines Against Burnout

Each presenter of the institute contributed suggestions and experiences to help practitioners continue their demanding work with AIDS clients and avoid burnout. The following is a summary of the insights and recommendations:

■ Persons with AIDS are warm, intelligent human beings, which makes relationships with these individuals enjoyable.

■ Use others as professional and personal reference groups to give you support.

■ Share feelings and maintain personal relationships with members of a specific support group.

■ Take time for yourself. Exercise, maintain interests, and keep active.

■ Get in touch with your feelings about AIDS and death.

■ Become familiar with the literature on death and dying and on suicide.

■ Become active in breaking boundaries between the systems that limit services provided to persons with AIDS.

■ Expect to move through a process in which you feel deep despair before you regain a more balanced sense of reality.

■ Use a voluntary system of staff rotation.

■ Staff might need to move to another area of practice with different clients and perhaps in different settings to use a different part of themselves.

CARL LEUKEFELD
MANUEL FIMBRES

March 1987

1

Statement of the Challenge

Caitlin C. Ryan

S ince the identification of AIDS in 1981, the syndrome, which has reached epidemic proportions, has become a central focus of social policy and practice. Across the country, we social workers—gay and straight, women and men, policy planners, group workers, community organizers, clinicians, welfare workers, and administrators—have emerged as leaders and innovators in developing programs, identifying resources, providing essential training and critical services, and building community-based AIDS organizations: the cornerstones of each community's response to the epidemic. Our unique training as advocates, facilitators, and enablers; our capacity to negotiate diverse systems; and our wide knowledge base have prompted us to deliver crucial services at a time when governmental leadership and interest have been noticeably absent and other groups have been paralyzed to respond.

Nevertheless, the efforts of social workers have been individual efforts. Such a personal response cannot address the profound social crisis generated by the AIDS epidemic. The capacity of the AIDS virus to lodge for years in the cell structure before emerging with overt symptomatology and the distressing level of ignorance that persists among the general public and health care professionals necessitate the immediate planning and implementation of a coordinated response to this crisis.

Our professional value base and the NASW Code of Ethics clearly dictate the need for an aggressive practice initiative. In particular, Section VI of the Code of Ethics mandates social work's responsibility to society during a time of public emergency and to minorities and oppressed groups who have been disproportionately affected by this epidemic. Although NASW has begun to deliberate policy issues related to AIDS, mounting an appropriate response requires the full support of NASW, the schools of social work, and leaders in all parts of the profession. Such a response should be generated initially through the association's network; the National Center for Social Policy and Practice should then begin to develop a comprehensive policy-practice model.

Incidence

As of September 11, 1986, more than 24,600 full-blown cases of AIDS have been reported to the Centers for Disease Control, an estimated 1.5 million individuals have already been exposed to the AIDS virus, and more than 13,600 individuals have died.[1] As Krim observed, "Americans in the prime of life are dying from AIDS at the rate of 200 each week and each week an even larger number of cases are diagnosed."[2]

Within the next five years, a dramatic increase in the incidence of AIDS is anticipated, which will require a widespread case management system that has yet to be designed. The chronic debilitating nature of the disease requires the development of intermediate care facilities, skilled nursing facilities, community care facilities, and additional services that would offer continuity of care to meet the essential needs of patients and to reduce the costs of hospitalization.

At the Coolfont conference in June 1986, 85 representatives of the U.S. Public Health Service (USPHS) and AIDS service programs estimated that by 1991, 145,000 individuals with AIDS will require medical care.[3] During that year, an additional 74,000 new cases will be diagnosed and 54,000 people will die. By the end of 1991, they anticipated that 270,000 cumulative cases of AIDS will have been reported. However, these figures may be at least 20 percent higher, given the tendency of some practitioners to underreport cases. According to current estimates of the rate of infection, more than 2.5 million persons could suffer from AIDS-related complex (20–30 percent of whom could develop AIDS), and 10 times that number could be infected with and capable of transmitting the virus.[4] At the Coolfont conference, the USPHS representatives acknowledged that they had clearly underestimated the velocity and threat of the epidemic so far—no surprise to the community organizations that have witnessed the great need for services and the intense concern of members of high-risk groups as well as the general public.

An increase in the number of heterosexually transmitted cases also is anticipated. Cases of heterosexual transmission now account for 7 percent of the cases, or approximately 1,100 reported cases. By 1991, this figure is projected to increase to 9 percent of the total, of 7,000 cases. In addition, by 1991 the number of children with AIDS, it is predicted, will be 10 times the current reported figure of 3,000.[5]

So far, cases of AIDS have been reported most frequently in major urban areas, with the greatest concentration in California and New York. By

1991, it is predicted that more than 80 percent of the cases will be reported from outside New York and San Francisco.[6] Yet, more jurisdictions and facilities wait until caseloads are pressing to implement services and to educate staff—a critical factor in ensuring appropriate services and the compliance of workers. In discussing the 40,000 cases predicted for 1991 in New York City alone, New York City's Commissioner of Health, Stephen Joseph, warned that the darkest days are still ahead of us.

Costs of Care

The costs of care will continue to escalate until comprehensive, coordinated, and community-oriented programs are organized to provide consistent case management. At the Coolfont conference, the USPHS representatives conservatively estimated that direct care costs for AIDS patients would reach $8–$16 billion by 1991, representing 1.2–2.4 percent of the total expenditures for personal health care in the United States.[7] Again, these figures could be underestimated by 10–50 percent because of the increased need for care of the large population of patients with other AIDS-related conditions and the significant nonmedical costs of managing these illnesses. In comparison, the cost of direct medical expenditures for the first 10,000 cases has been estimated at $1.4 billion.[8]

Hospital costs for AIDS patients are, on the average, 60–70 percent higher than for all other patients. For example, the Greater New York Hospital Association estimated that AIDS patients require two to three times more care from nursing staff than do other patients and that their need for psychological support is greater.[9] As the number of indigent and uninsured patients with AIDS increases, as it surely will, the amount of revenue lost in the treatment of the average AIDS patient ("uncollectibles") will threaten the quality of care these patients can receive within a profit-driven health care system. Stephen Gamble, president of the Hospital Council of Southern California, estimated that the uncollectibles for an AIDS patient are 3.4 times higher than those for the average non-AIDS patient.[10] Outside the hospital setting, reimbursement is poor for long-term care, including hospices, although hospices are the most effective, cost-efficient, and humane services for dying AIDS patients.

Through the careful planning and coordination of services, and the cooperation and mobilization of diverse social groups, systems, and institutions, these problems can be addressed and resolved. The social response to AIDS was initiated and carried out by the gay community through the development and funding of community-based AIDS service organizations, and much of the expertise in managing AIDS is concentrated in this minority group. However, new alliances and coalitions must be formed to share knowledge and information, and new systems must evolve to address the continuing problems of serving chronically ill patients. As the report concluded, the response to AIDS must be broadened to "reflect the pluralistic character of the American health care system and must involve the coordinated participation of the public, private, and voluntary sectors as well as ambulatory, in-hospital, and long-term care providers."[11]

Barriers to the Provision of Services

Certainly, more than the large number of cases and the unresponsive health care delivery system are impeding the delivery of services. Pervasive homophobia, coupled with the growing public phobia about AIDS, has inhibited a rapid response and the development of a national campaign to educate the public about AIDS. Without effective treatment and the potential for a vaccine still years away, prevention is imperative. Not only would a national education program reduce the risk of AIDS among uninfected individuals, it would defuse the fear of AIDS by the general public and encourage a more compassionate response to friends or co-workers who are diagnosed with AIDS. However, given the current political climate for social and health services, it is unlikely that such an educational program will be instituted either by the federal government or by a professional association. This is an area in which social work systems, institutions, and practitioners are capable of providing an essential service—once materials and information have been made available to all service providers—through a nationally coordinated social work response. NASW must take the leadership role in initiating this response. In early 1986, an AIDS action plan was introduced to the NASW Board of Directors, based on the NASW Public Policy statement on AIDS that was adopted by the Delegate Assembly in 1984. Action on that plan is pending.[12]

Concerns over AIDS-related discrimination have emerged as a central focus for discussing the rights of society versus the rights of individuals. Many of the rights of AIDS patients to employment, housing, confidentiality, and care have been dealt with and will continue to be addressed through the courts. A recent U.S. Department of Justice opinion, that the Federal Rehabilitation Act's prohibition of discrimination against handicapped people does not apply to individuals with AIDS if an employer is afraid that AIDS could be spread in the workplace, flies in the face of consistent medical evidence that AIDS is not casually spread.[13] The American Medical Association opposed this opinion,[14] and many state and local jurisdictions have overlooked it, relying instead on available scientific data to support the rights of patients. As an article in the *Harvard Law Review* stated: "Unfortunately, AIDS-control laws may be enacted in response to public misconceptions about transmission of the virus and inappropriate assumptions about the moral culpability of its victims."[15]

Furthermore, in earlier epidemics, public health regulations restricted the rights of individuals. As the aforementioned article noted:

> Courts' treatment of public health regulation has changed very little since the turn of the century. Although in the 1920's courts began to

require some showing of medical necessity as the science of public health advanced, they continued to allow class membership alone to justify public health restrictions when a disfavored class, such as prostitutes, was the subject of the regulation. These judicial opinions assumed that victims were to blame for their illnesses. The attitude that the diseased are a "menace" to both health and morals survived through the 1950's and 1960's, when incarcerated tuberculosis patients challenged state authority to quarantine; such an attitude could easily reappear when AIDS cases come to court.[16]

Compulsory testing, the violation of confidentiality, and quarantine are critical issues in addressing discrimination against AIDS patients. As client advocates, social workers increasingly will be required to intervene to protect the rights of clients and to explain procedures and rights to clients and their families. The potential for societal descrimination against vulnerable groups clearly exists. The overwhelming concentration of AIDS cases among minorities has tipped the scales away from an early well-organized effort to end the epidemic. Ironically, by denying that *anyone* may be at risk of being infected with AIDS, as has been done because of prejudicial attitudes about "high-risk" groups and the resultant failure to provide timely education about prevention, the number of at-risk groups has increased exponentially.

Conclusion

Social workers have a vital role to play in the AIDS crisis, and our leadership in determining social policies, in conducting research about its social consequences, in developing services, in training, and in planning curricula is essential. Every relevant social issue of our time is raised in relation to AIDS. If we searched for a more powerful agent of social change, we would never find it.

The AIDS crisis is perhaps the greatest opportunity in this century to incorporate the values of our profession—respect for differences, self-determination for all individuals, the rights to confidentiality and privacy, the commitment to community service, ethical responsibility to society—within the institutions that govern us. Perhaps the greatest hidden struggle of the epidemic—the political and professional "ownership" of the AIDS crisis—is one in which social work must remain centrally involved. Who represents us and how our views are articulated and woven into the developing policies and services in an emerging field of practice are critical issues in the delivery of high-quality humane services to clients and the responsiveness of the health care system.

The emerging problems of AIDS are clearly social and ethical problems—not merely clinical problems. They pose a pivotal challenge to which the social work profession must unite and respond.

Notes and References

1. "AIDS Weekly Surveillance Report" (Atlanta, Ga.: Centers for Disease Control, September 11, 1986), p. 1.

2. M. Krim, "Editorial on AZT," *New York Times,* 24 (August 1986).

3. "Coolfont Report: A PHS Plan for Prevention and Control of AIDS and the AIDS Virus," *Public Health Reports,* 101 (July–August 1986), pp. 342–343.

4. "Future Shock," *Newsweek,* 24 (November 1986), p. 30.

5. "Coolfont Report," p. 343.

6. Ibid.

7. Ibid., p. 348.

8. D. Holtzman, "New AIDS Victim: Hospital Budgets," *Insight,* 25 (August 1986), p. 54.

9. Ibid.

10. Ibid.

11. "Coolfont Report," p. 348.

12. C. Ryan and L. Caputo, "AIDS at the Interface: Policy, Practice and Social Change." Invitational paper presented at the NASW Professional Symposium, Chicago, 1985.

13. R. Pear, "Justice Department Rights Laws Offer Only Limited Help on AIDS, U.S. Rules," *New York Times,* 23 (June 1986), p. 1.

14. S. Okie, "AMA Opposes Justice Department on AIDS Bias," *Washington Post,* 11 (July 1986), p. 1.

15. "Constitutional Rights of AIDS Carriers," *Harvard Law Review,* 99 (April 1986), p. 1274.

16. Ibid., p. 1277

2

Current and Anticipated Trends

Carl G. Leukefeld and Robert J. Battjes

This article presents an overview of selected trends related to AIDS with an emphasis on issues relevant to social workers.[1] Many people, including social workers, are asking such general questions as, "Where did AIDS come from, and how can the spread of this fatal disease be so rapid? Why was AIDS not known about years ago, and how can the infection process be prevented?" Parallels are drawn to the Black Plague and to tuberculosis. In other arenas, the focus is on the politics of allocating resources and on those groups that have been affected by AIDS.

The answers to these questions are not dealt with here, but they set the stage for this discussion because they are the most obvious questions about AIDS. AIDS is a behavior-driven disease in that most persons are exposed to the virus that causes AIDS by engaging in specific risk behaviors. Social work has concentrated on the behavioral aspects of disease from the days of Mary Richmond to the present, and social workers have identified the coping strategies and skills that individuals as well as families need to deal with crises in their lives. Clearly, AIDS is an important, if not the major, public health issue in this country and in many other parts of the world today. Furthermore, on the basis of current knowledge, AIDS will remain a major public health issue for many years to come because no vaccine is available to prevent the disease and it will be years before a vaccine or drugs to treat AIDS will be developed.

The AIDS Virus

The human immunodeficiency virus (HIV)—the virus that causes AIDS—belongs to a family of retroviruses known for more than 50 years to cause leukemias, lymphomas, and immune deficiency conditions in animals. Other human retroviruses include the adult T-cell leukemia virus. A major characteristic of retroviruses is their incorporation into the T-4 cells, and they are reproduced every time an infected cell divides. T-4 cells are helper cells that direct other T cells and B cells that recognize foreign matter so the T-8 (suppressor cells) can destroy the invaded cells.

The AIDS virus attacks the immune system, causing a range of immunologic disturbances that make a person susceptible to opportunistic infections and cancers. A diagnosis of AIDS requires the presence of one or more opportunistic diseases indicative of underlying cellular immunodeficiency in the absence of known causes of underlying reduced immunity. These opportunistic diseases include protozoan infections, fungal infections, bacterial infections, noncongenital viral infections, certain cancers, and helminthic infection. The most common opportunistic diseases that are characteristic of AIDS are pneumocystis carinii pneumonia and Kaposi's sarcoma. In addition to attacking the immune system, the HIV also attacks the brain, producing neurological disorders that, in some instances, precede the onset of clinical AIDS.

Until recently, persons with AIDS could be treated for specific opportunistic diseases, but there was no treatment for the underlying immunodeficiency. The experimental drug azidothymidine (AZT) has now been shown to halt the replication of the AIDS virus with some manifestations of AIDS. Although AZT is able to prolong the lives of persons with AIDS, it is not a cure for the syndrome.

It is important to distinguish HIV infections from AIDS itself. The vast majority of individuals who are infected with the AIDS virus are apparently healthy, and it is unclear how many will eventually contract AIDS. Infected individuals may remain healthy for years but later develop the disease (the median time lag between infection and disease is estimated to be four years). Yet, asymptomatic infected individuals unknowingly are able to transmit the virus to others.

The Spread of AIDS

According to estimates from the USPHS, 1 million to 1.5 million Americans were infected with HIV as of June 1986. Although it is not clear how many of these people will eventually develop AIDS, current data suggest that 20–30 percent of those who are now infected will develop AIDS by the end of 1991. Thus, is it expected that, by the end of 1991, 270,000 individuals will meet the surveillance definition of AIDS by the Centers for Disease Control. Medical costs are projected to reach $8–16 billion by that time.[2]

As Table 1 indicates, the USPHS projection is that an estimated 35,000 persons will have been diagnosed with AIDS by the end of 1986, with 16,000 new cases in that year alone. With this projection comes the grim expectation that the annual death rate will continue to rise until it reaches 54,000 in 1991, when the cumulative total of deaths is projected to be 179,000.

Table 1. Projected Cases of AIDS in the United States[a]

Category	1986	1991	1991 Range
Cases Diagnosed			
Cumulative cases at the start of the year	19,000	196,000	155,000–220,000
Diagnosed during the year	16,000	74,000	46,000– 91,000
Alive at the start of the year	10,000	71,000	50,000– 83,000
Alive during the year	26,000	145,000	96,000–180,000
Deaths			
Cumulative deaths at the start of the year	9,000	125,000	103,000–137,000
Deaths during the year	9,000	54,000	37,000– 64,000
Cumulative deaths at the end of the year	18,000	179,000	142,000–201,000
Infections			
Persons with HTLV-III/ LAV infection	1,000,000 to 1,500,000 (estimate)		

[a]These numbers refer only to those cases that meet the definition of AIDS by the Centers for Disease Control (*see Morbidity and Mortality Weekly Report,* 34 (1985, pp. 373–375) and do not include other manifestations of infection, such as AIDS-related complex and lymphadenopathy syndrome.

Source: "Coolfont Report: A PHS Plan for Prevention and Control of AIDS and the AIDS Virus," *Public Health Reports,* 101 (July–August 1986), pp. 343–348.

Prevalence of AIDS

Table 2 indicates that cases of AIDS are most prevalent in five standard metropolitan statistical areas in the United States, which generally are located on the East and West coasts and that the New York City area has the largest number of persons with AIDS. Whereas New York City and San Francisco now account for 42 percent of cases of AIDS, it is anticipated that by 1991, only 20 percent of the cases will be from these two cities because the disease will have spread by then to other parts of the country.[3]

Tables 3 through 6 present the demographic characteristics of persons with AIDS. The total number of AIDS cases from 1981 to May 5, 1986, was 20,016. The largest at-risk group are homosexual/bisexual men, who constitute 73 percent of all AIDS cases; intravenous drug users also constitute 11 percent of this group. The second largest at-risk group (17 percent of all cases) is heterosexual intravenous drug users. Because 11 percent of the homosexual/bisexual cases (or 8 percent of all adult cases) have used drugs intravenously, intravenous drug users make up 25 percent of all persons with AIDS. Table 4 indicates that 60 percent of the persons with AIDS are white, 25 percent are black, 14 percent are Hispanic, and 1 percent are from other racial or ethnic groups of are persons whose racial/ethnic group is unknown.

Table 2. Reported Cases of AIDS, by Standard Metropolitan Statistical Area (SMSA) of Residence, 1981 to May 5, 1986

SMSA of Residence	Cases	Percentage of Total Cases	Cases per 1 Million Population[a]
New York City	6,288	31	689.4
San Francisco	2,144	11	659.6
Miami	604	3	371.5
Newark	507	2	257.9
Los Angeles	1,737	9	232.3
Elsewhere in the United States	9,025	44	44.2
Total	20,305	100	

[a]The Centers for Disease Control derived the *Cases per 1 Million Population* category from the 1980 census. The case rate per million for the total U.S. population is 89.2.

Source: Centers for Disease Control, May 1986.

Table 3. Reported Cases of Adults with AIDS, by Risk Group, United States, 1981 to May 5, 1986 (N = 20,016)

Risk Group	Percentage
Homosexual/bisexual men[a]	73
Intravenous drug users	17
Persons with hemophilia coagulation disorder	1
Heterosexual who had contact with infected persons	1
Persons who received a transfusion with blood or blood products	2
Others/unknown	6

[a]Eleven percent of the homosexual/bisexual males reported having used intravenous drugs.

Source: Centers for Disease Control, May 1986.

Table 4. Reported Cases of AIDS by Racial/Ethnic Group, United States, 1981 to May 5, 1986

Racial/Ethnic Groups	Cases	Percentage of Total
White	12,067	60
Black	5,106	25
Hispanic	2,903	14
Other/unknown	229	1
Total	20,305	100

Source: Centers for Disease Control, May 1986.

Table 5. Reported Cases of AIDS, by Age Group, United States, 1981 to May 5, 1986

Age Groups	Cases	Percentage of Total
Less than 13 years	289	1
13–19 years	84	0
20–29 years	4,248	21
30–39 years	9,529	47
40–49 years	4,211	21
Over 49 years	1,944	10
Total	20,305	100

Source: Centers for Disease Control, May 1986.

Table 6. Cases of Children with AIDS, by Risk Group, May 5, 1986 (*N* = 289)

Risk Groups	Percentage of Total
Children with a hemophilia/coagulation disorder	4
Children whose parent has AIDS or is at increased risk of contracting AIDS	76
Children who received a transfusion with blood or blood products	15
Others/unknown	5

Source: Centers for Disease Control, May 1986.

Table 5 shows that persons with AIDS are young; 47 percent are aged 30–39 years, and only 10 percent are over 49 years. Table 6 indicates that over three-fourths (76 percent) of the 289 children with AIDS have parents who have AIDS or parents who are at an increased risk of contracting AIDS.

Transmission and Prevention of AIDS

The Centers for Disease Control have found that the AIDS virus can be transmitted in a number of different ways. Specific routes of the transmission of HIV include sex (homosexual sex between men or heterosexual sex—with transmission occuring from men to women and women to men), exposure to blood (the sharing of needles by drug users; the transfusion of blood, plasma, packed cells platelets, and factor concentrates; and occupational injuries from needle pricks), and perinatal (prepartum, intrapartum, and possibly postpartum).

It is important for social workers to have information about how AIDS may be prevented so they may provide the information to their clients. The USPHS provides six recommendations for preventing the spread of AIDS:

1. Individuals should not have sex with persons who have AIDS, who are infected with HIV, or who are at an increased risk of contracting AIDS. In addition, they should not have sex with multiple partners or with persons who have had multiple partners.

2. Individuals should not give blood if they are at risk of contracting AIDS.

3. Health workers should use extreme care when handling or disposing of hypodermic needles.

4. Individuals should not abuse intravenous drugs. Those who use intravenous drugs should not share needles or syringes.

5. Women who use intravenous drugs or are sexual partners of members of risk groups should consider the risk of transmission to unborn babies before they become pregnant.

6. Individuals should not use inhalant nitrites (poppers), because they may play a role as a cofactor in Kaposi's sarcoma.

For persons with positive HIV antibody tests, the USPHS suggests the following to prevent the spread of AIDS: have regular medical evaluations and follow-ups; do not donate blood, plasma, body organs, other tissue, or sperm; and take precautions against exchanging body fluids during sexual activity.

Because vaccines to prevent the spread of AIDS are not available, methods to control AIDS are directed toward behavioral change and voluntary serological testing, accompanied by appropriate counseling. Serological testing determines whether a person is infected with HIV—not whether a person has or will contract AIDS. Testing should include an initial screening with the enzyme-linked immunosorbent assay test and a confirmation of positive tests by a more specific methods such as Western blot. It is recommended that testing be voluntary and be accompanied by both pre- and posttest counseling regarding the meaning of the test results and risk-reduction measures.

Intravenous drug users constitute one of the two groups at highest risk of contracting AIDS.[4] Among intravenous drug users, AIDS is spread largely through sharing needles with other addicts, which results in a high seroprevalence of HIV, which, in turn, leads to the development of AIDS in this population. The prevalence of HIV seropositivity among homosexual men and intravenous drug users parallels the frequency of AIDS in various cities.[5] In addition, homosexual/bisexual men and men and women who use drugs intravenously will continue to be the populations at highest risk for HIV infection for the next five years. Therefore, strategies to deal with drug abuse, as well as the sexual practices of homosexual and bisexual men, must be developed if the spread of the AIDS epidemic is to be halted. Three specific areas to be emphasized are these: (1) the number of intravenous drug users in treatment must be increased, (2) the effectiveness of treatment programs must be improved so that relapse becomes less common, and (3) information and other interventions that are designed to change risk-related behaviors must be provided so that the likelihood is significantly reduced that the disease will spread among intravenous drug users and from them to their sexual partners and children.

Conclusion

The trend data presented here provide a frame of reference for social work services. Clearly, AIDS has spread and will continue to spread dramatically into all segments of the population in the next few years. In the absence of effective vaccines to prevent AIDS and drugs to treat it, social workers have an important role to play in helping individuals and their loved ones to plan for and cope with impending death and those at risk of contracting AIDS to modify their behavior. Just as social work's core values and knowledge base have guided the profession in addressing various challenges throughout its history, they will enable the profession to respond to the current challenge of AIDS.

Notes and References

1. Incidence and prevalence data cited in this article are from the Centers for Disease Control, Atlanta, Georgia, as of 1986.

2. "Coolfont Report: A PHS Plan for Prevention and Control of AIDS and the AIDS Virus," *Public Health Reports,* 101 (July–August 1986), p. 348.

3. Ibid., p. 343.

4. "AIDS and the IV Drug Abuser: Strategies for Combating the Epidemic." Unpublished report of the Technical Review Conference (Rockville, Md.: National Institute on Drug Abuse, July 1986).

5. "Coolfont Report."

3

Research on the Psychosocial Aspects of AIDS: A Review

Martin Schwartz

Research on AIDS has focused predominately on the identification of the HTLV-III virus, the transmission of the virus through blood and semen products, and the demographics of high-risk behaviors. Despite the biopsychosocial aspects of the disease, it only has been recently that researchers have responded to the concerns of practitioners with people who have AIDS about the lack of data on the psychological and social realities of persons with AIDS and AIDS-related complex (ARC). Practitioners have recognized that educational and preventive programs may not be providing the most appropriate content because they have been based not on data but on the public health ideology used in the past with other public health issues. Learning more about the sociocultural context of AIDS and ARC, their clinical course, and the interrelationship of the environment and the neuroendocrine immune system are more effective means of obtaining data on which information, treatment, and public policy could be developed.

This article synthesizes the current empirical data on the psychosocial aspects of AIDS and ARC and highlights the impact of the research on programs for persons with AIDS and ARC. It follows the classification system of psychosocial studies identified at the 1984 workshop of the Institute of the Advancement of Health: (1) *onset studies,* which deal with pre-existing traits characteristic of high-risk behavior and stress related to gay life and the AIDS epidemic; and (2) *psychological needs studies,* which center on the responses of persons with AIDS and ARC. Included within the latter category are research on coping styles, clinical evidence of maladaptation, and the impact of social support systems.[1]

Obstacles to Research

It is important to assess the geopolitical environment in which psychosocial studies on AIDS have been conducted to understand the inherent limitations of doing research in an atmosphere of devastating negative policies, attitudes, and behaviors toward persons with AIDS and ARC. AIDS was first reported to the Centers for Disease Control in 1981 by a young California physician, Dr. Michael Gottleib, who described a new lethal illness that was striking young men in their prime. Gottlieb's findings were echoed by others who were seeing young men with such strange symptoms of opportunistic diseases as pneumocystic carinii pneumonia, the purple lesions of Kaposi's sarcoma, the ulcerated mouth and throat of cadia albicans, and severe diarrhea caused by exotic bacteria. In 1981, 225 cases were reported. In May 1983, a French team published evidence of a new virus that played a significant role in the etiology of the syndrome. In spring 1984, the National Cancer Institute announced that the AIDS virus had been conclusively identified.[2] On June 13, 1986, *The New York Times* reported that 21,517 cases of AIDS and 11,713 deaths were recorded by the government. Projections for the future are that by 1991, there will be a cumulative total of 270,000 cases and 179,000 deaths.[3]

Accurate incidence and prevalence rates still are difficult to ascertain because of the narrow definition of AIDS by the Centers for Disease Control, the refusal by some physicians to list AIDS on death certificates, and the wide variation in the incubation period of the illness. Although AIDS has been found in heterosexual men and women, it was first named gay-related immune deficiency because the highest percentage (73 percent) of reported cases were gay and bisexual men.[4]

Because of its unique characteristics and the reactions to the disease, AIDS has become a challenge and a threat to the medical profession, the public health sector, the public welfare sector, the legal system, and the moral fiber of our society. It continues to pose a public health threat because there still is no positive test for AIDS (the test shows only the presence of antibodies) and no cure or prophylaxis to prevent one from being infected by the virus. Moreover, societal attitudes have compounded the personal tragedy for those who are afflicted with AIDS or ARC by stigmatizing, isolating, and rejecting them. The threat to the civil rights of persons with AIDS and ARC still is great—in the form of proposed quarantine camps, denial of insurance coverage, denial of protection from job discrimination, and the loss of schooling and housing. The fact that the initial victims of the AIDS epidemic in the United States have been gay men and intravenous drug users has permitted the more virulent and maleficent attitudes and behaviors to dictate the public's and government's responses to the epidemic. Persons with AIDS are the lepers of the 1980s.

Homophobia

An inherent difficulty in researching the gay population in this country is that its prevalence is still shrouded with unknowns because of homophobia, stigma, and possible disenfranchisement, as illustrated by the "Supreme Court decision to endorse Georgia's right to declare sodomy a crime [which rejected] the argument that such a law invades privacy and strikes at deeply personal, basic liberties."[5] Researchers must be cognizant of the defensiveness of the gay population, since the scientific literature is replete with slanderous descriptions of perverted, drug-taking, hedonistic, and sexually promiscuous gay men.[6]

Because the precise number of gay men is not known, researchers have no way of enumerating the population for sampling reliabilty and validity. Joseph et al. argued that one solution is to define a probability sample and use it only as a subpopulation.[7] Thus, one can cover many subpopulations for an association of findings yet be cautious about the applicability of the findings to all gays. Bradford found that the degree of "outness" affected changes in behavior and attitudes.[8] Again, the varying of degrees of "outness" and "closetedness" are just too loose to be applied across the boards when one considers geographic differences, age, and the changing views of the political-legal systems about homosexuality.

Furthermore, as Joseph urged, researchers should be compassionate toward and knowledgeable about the mores and cultures of all the populations that are at risk of contracting AIDS.[9] These attitudes are especially important in relation to gays.

Moreover, it has been pointed out that researchers have to understand the complex significance of medical advice to gays.[10] Before the AIDS epidemic, "gay sex" was considered to be against nature—now it is life threatening. Therefore, medical presciptions can be perceived by gay men as affirmations of the legitimacy of homophobic attitudes. Coates, Temoshok, and Mandel eloquently crystallized the dilemma as follows:

> The connection between sex behavior and fear of death and damnation is a theme rooted in our Judeo-Christian traditions, our laws and our social structure. For gay persons, this connection almost invariably includes social stigma and the potential for oppression. With the advent of AIDS, sex and affectional love between men is associated strongly with the transmission of a potentially lethal agent.[11]

Homophobic responses have influenced the international scientific community and have blocked cooperation in identifying the course of the virus. Determining accurate reactions to AIDS in places like Turkana, where people show no symptoms of AIDS but evidence infection of the virus, is important because somehow they may have developed an immunity to the disease. "Clearly, no country really wants to learn it is the original source of AIDS. Countries have been playing a game of geographical buck passing with each other, each citing the other as a source."[12] The finding of AIDS in heterosexuals may be the reason for the World Health Organization's decision in November 1986 to mount a global campaign to control the disease.

Racism

As one peruses the literature, it becomes obvious that, in research, AIDS and ARC are still synonymous with gay white men. Caputo pointed out that those intravenous drug abusers who develop AIDS and ARC are primarily people of color and women.[13] Gilberto Gerald, executive director of the National Coalition of Black Gays, bemoaned:

> The popular and wide-spread conception is that AIDS is a disorder affecting white males. While it is true that 71% are classified as homosexual/bisexual, it is also true that 26% of these gay males are Black, 14% are Hispanic and 40% of the persons with AIDS overall are of the Third World Extraction. Many drug users, who constitute 17% of all persons with AIDS, are also Black, Hispanic or Gay.[14]

Gerald and others have decried the lack of research geared toward this population and have warned that public agencies and AIDS-related service organizations need to evaluate, continually monitor, and improve the effectiveness of their programs with regard to the impact on the Third World gay community if we are going to win the war against AIDS.[15]

Psychosocial studies reported in the literature have acknowledged the serious limitation just described—that most of the data are on gay white men.[16] One certainly could infer that racism is just as prevalent in the gay population as it is the "straight" population. The lack of data may also indicate that the health care system is not as accessible to nonwhites as it is to whites. Furthermore, despite attempts by some researchers to include people of color as participants, one needs to ask whether the color and ethnicity of researchers is a significant variable of the failures of studies to tap the nonwhite population.

Finally, it has been noted that persons with ARC have been understudied because of their lack of involvement in programs for AIDS.[17] To omit this cohort is to overlook a significant number of people and to lose the opportunity to gain much-needed information about coping and stress.

Onset Studies

Onset studies examine the impact of psychological experiences on health. Most studies draw on the framework of psychoneuroimmunology, which investigates connections between psychological factors, neurological mediators, and immune status.[18] The assumption is that, as is true in relation to other diseases, internal and external stress will influence a person's susceptibility to AIDS and contribute to health-promoting or health-damaging behavior. In addition, the studies acknowledge that coping "is not a coherent, stable and linear series of responses to threat. Instead it is more often an inconsistent shifting and related set of cognitions and behaviors. Decisions made at one point are modified later by experiences and new information."[19]

Some onset studies attempt to define the individual's host vulnerability to the virus through research based on "interactive models." These models present a paradigm of factors that are relevant to the body's ability to resist the disease when exposed to it that go beyond agents and substances to a broad range of behavioral, social, and psychological criteria, including the community.[20] Although studies are being conducted to identify psychosocial variables that operate as cofactors to immunocompetence and to elucidate the connections between these variables, most published studies have explored the sexual behavior of identified high-risk populations to determine whether these groups have reduced their risky sexual practices and undergone any concomitant psychological reactions.

Findings

Gattozzi found that, in general,

> rapid and substantial changes have been made by the majority of study subjects in many aspects of sexual behavior considered to be risk factors for AIDS. Nevertheless, a significant proportion of the subjects continued to engage in sexual behavior and specific practices considered to be unsafe.[21]

More specifically, a follow-up study in San Francisco in 1985 found a continued substantial reduction of risky sexual practices by gays, both with long-term partners and with strangers, and an increase in safe sex practices.[22] Yet, one fourth of the entire cohort of 361 reported engaging in at least one sexual act capable of infecting themselves and 28.4 percent stated that they have engaged in a sexual act with a stranger that could have infected others with the virus. These men sometimes chose to abstain from sexual activity rather than to move from high-risk practices to low-risk practices. Four variables distinguished those who reduced the number of their sexual partners: an ability to recall an image of someone who had deteriorated from AIDS, younger age, having a primary relationship, and being newer to gay life. A greater use of denial was found in those men who engaged in practices that were capable of either transmitting or receiving the virus.

In New York City, Martin found that the documented declines in the percentages of those engaging in specific sexual practices were not translating into equally large proportions of men who were reducing their risk of exposure to the virus.[23] In other words, gay men in New York City may be acknowledging specific aspects of risky practices without attending to all the risk factors simultaneously. In Chicago, Joseph et al. found that the factors that were predictive of future behavioral change included the years of the homosexual experience, a knowledge of risk factors, and the availability of social support.[24] Men who changed had greater perceptions of their vulnerability to contract AIDS and an ability to handle the stress associated with limiting the number of their sexual partners. Siegel indicated that although all the conditions of the health-belief model were met by nearly all the study subjects, which would lead one to predict their adoption of safe sexual practices, many continued to engage in risky practices with multiple partners.[25] The preliminary findings of Puchall and Van Ness's study in Washington, D.C., support the idea that most people make rational changes but that a large minority does not.[26]

Psychosocial studies have underscored the stress experienced by gay men because of the AIDS epidemic and the imminence of death. Most gay men report intense feelings of despair, distress, and fear owing to the revitalization of antigay feelings and threats of quarantine and other punitive measures to isolate. The effects of chronic stress (decreased levels of energy, concentration, and restful sleep) were seen in a sample of more than 5,000 asymptomatic at-risk men in four cities (Baltimore, Chicago, Los Angeles, and Pittsburgh).[27] Although may gay men have adopted safer sexual practices, they may already have been exposed to the deadly virus. Medical education efforts do not seem to be addressing the cost of change in sexual behavior to the psyches of gay men, such as the "sense of betrayal of one's identity and one's subcultural norms."[28]

One needs to be cognizant that, to survive, gay men must make changes in the most intimate, symbolic, and idiosyncratic human condition: sex. They need to accept that the information they receive is not another attempt by the straight world to inhibit the behavior that makes them different. Furthermore, they must make changes now—even if their past sexual history has already endangered their lives. The uncertainty of their situation, caused by the long incubation period for AIDS and the lack of an accurate diagnosis until the telltale symptoms appear, further complicates the decision-making process. The lifestyles of some gay men, which have provided them with an identity and membership in a group, now are being questioned. To some, the changes would equal estrangement or isolation; to all, the aesthetics and pleasures of sexuality now are contaminated. Moreover, as is the case with any threat to one's existence, there will be some who need to deny their vulnerability or emphasize their superhuman ability not to be infected, no matter what practices they engage in.

The reported studies emphasize the need for community support programs that will promote safe sex and the idea that gays must control their lives by taking responsibility for not harming themselves or others. Models of gay men are needed to provide positive leadership and to symbolize healthy coping strategies for dealing with the stress-related changes in sexual practices. Support groups identify alternative ways, other than bars and bathhouses, for gays to meet, to be intimate, and to support each other. Moreover, it is critical that gays concentrate on building physical and psychological resistance to deal with the challenge of the virus to the immune system. As Bradford suggested, coming out of the closet and making connections with other gays through social activism (such as campaigns to revoke sodomy laws) can be another channel for developing the positive identity needed to offset external stressors.[29]

Psychological Needs Studies

Psychological needs studies explore the changed psychological and social situations of individuals who have contracted AIDS or ARC. Related studies similarly examine the psychosocial needs of high-risk populations. The aim of some studies is to develop and evaluate interventions to meet the psychosocial needs of such groups.[30] All the studies have agreed that the persons with AIDS respond to their fate as others have responded to life-threatening illnesses—with anxiety, distress, and depression—and that they go through the same stages of anticipatory grief (denial, anger, bargaining, depression, and acceptance) noted by Kübler-Ross.[31] The findings of many studies of the psychological responses of the gay populations reflect Holland's findings that 79 percent of the ARC group, 59 percent of the AIDS group, and 41 percent of the gay-bisexual "worried well" group had diagnoses on Axis I of the *Diagnostic and Statistical Manual of Mental Disorders (Third Edition)*—depression or adjustment reaction with depression.[32] One consistent finding that has been difficult to understand fully is that ARC groups show the highest distress and depression; most researchers infer that the psychological responses of persons with ARC stem from a fear of the "unknown" and an "anticipation" of what will happen to them.[33]

The human experiences and feelings beneath the statistics reflect the impact of homophobia on persons with AIDS and ARC. For example, individuals report that they do not disclose their medical problems or symptoms to professionals or to their families for fear that they would then be sentenced to an isolated death.[34] Researchers report that the persons with ARC and AIDS project their unfortunate fate onto their gayness—that the disease is a retribution for their sexual proclivity.[35] Persons with ARC and AIDS are disillusioned and angry at the lack of effective treatment and the discrimination that usually accompanies the diagnosis. The degradation, the variety of dehumanizing experiences, the pain, and the lack of hope have led many to consider suicide. Support groups, as well as the recent more receptive attitudes of some medical professionals who are willing to diagnose and treat patients with AIDS, have proved successful in neutralizing some of these psychological responses. Dreher reported studies of different approaches to groups that teach structured coping strategies, emotional support, and relaxation techniques.[36] It is evident that the goals of social support groups are to replace lost friends and family, reduce the stigmatization of AIDS, and help persons with AIDS and ARC gain some control over their lives, helping them to regain their self-esteem. To achieve these goals with the worried well and persons with ARC is to aid their survival.

As Perry and Jacobson indicated,

> . . . psychiatric symptoms among patients with AIDS may be functional reactions to contracting a fatal and stigmatizing disease or may be secondary to malignancies and opportunistic infections on the central nervous system. More recent evidence indicates that HTLV-III directly infects the central nervous system and may cause psychiatric symptoms.[37]

They reported that such mental syndromes may mimic functional disorders and may appear before signs of immunodeficiency or neurological signs emerge. Therefore, they emphasized the need for vigilance in detecting organic impairment through periodic neurological and neuropsychological examinations of persons with ARC and individuals whose serum contains the HTLV-III according to the Western blot test.

The paradoxes of AIDS may be symbolized by the confusion and the consequences of the confusion surrounding testing for AIDS. Immunologists have agreed that HTLV-III is a presumptive etiological agent in the pathogenesis of AIDS. Most will accept that HTLV-III is a "marker for AIDS, and its diagnostic and medical applications should not be suspended."[38] However, the public needs to understand that a positive antibody test does not prove the presence of the virus and, furthermore, that the presence of an active virus does not prove the inevitability of contracting AIDS or ARC. The ELISA test has been found to produce "about six percent of false positive results."[39] The Western blot test is considered to be more reliable yet recent data shows a much higher rate of both "false positives" and "false negatives" than was expected.[40]

Another complication of the testing is that insurance companies and employers are insisting on using the test to weed out persons who may have AIDS or to deny them hospitalization and death benefits. Although public officials have enacted laws to protect the confidentiality of the testees, Raskin speculated that "it will be tempting for public health officials and courts to forget the rights of infected people; yet individuals' rights must not be ignored or glossed over as we meet the scientific challenges ahead."[41] Thus, anyone who takes a test for AIDS faces the loss of confidentiality, an ambiguity about the accuracy of the results, and a possible "death sentence." Researchers are attempting to obtain clearer pictures of psychological adaptations that occur from taking the test. Speculation ranges from the idea that just taking the test could be enough of a stressor to overload the immune system to the obvious idea of the need for counseling before and after testing by self-help groups, which AIDS programs have utilized as effective community support interventions.

Although psychosocial factors in AIDS and ARC have been underresearched, there are indications that many studies are in progress.[42] Indeed, data reported here may be obsolete. Researchers are investigating the adaptation of persons with AIDS who have lived beyond the estimated two years. They are seeking answers to the differences in the psychoneuroimmunologic systems of men with high-risk behavior who become infected with AIDS and ARC and those who do not and are evaluating the efficacy of prevention programs geared toward changing high-risk behavior to low-risk behavior. However, the impact of AIDS and ARC on other populations—people of color, women, and intravenous drug users—still needs to be determined. And as AIDS and ARC move into the heterosexual populations in this country, it is obvious that attention to these populations will be mandatory as well.

AIDS is an illness of national, if not international proportions, that encompasses health, legal, and familial issues, as well as the victim's person-in-situation. It is a personal tragedy excaberated by negative societal attitudes. AIDS is John, whose mother and wife had to find a meatpacker to embalm him so he could be buried. AIDS is Phil, who had to expose his tongue and throat to his employer so the employer could determine if Phil was infected. AIDS is Carl, who checks his body each night for the telltale purple lesions and waits for the inevitable time bomb to explode within him and destroy his virile young body. It is these images that we researchers must engrave in our consciousness as we research this devastating plague of the 1980s and 1990s.

Notes and References

1. H. Dreher, "The Psychosocial Aspects of AIDS," Summary of the Workshop of the Institute of the Advancement of Health, 1984.

2. N. Meredith, "The Gay Dilemma," *Psychology Today* (Jaunary 1984), pp. 55–62.

3. Robert Pear, "Tenfold Increase in AIDS Death Toll is Expected by '91," *New York Times,* June 13, 1986, pp. 1 and 11.

4. J. Lang, J. Spiegel, and S. Strigle, *Living with AIDS—A Self-Care Manual* (West Hollywood, Calif.: AIDS Project Los Angeles, 1985).

5. Editorial, *New York Times,* June 23, 1986, p. A22.

6. W. F. Batchelor, "AIDS: A Public Health and Psychological Emergency," *American Psychologist,* 39 (November 1984), pp. 1279–1284.

7. J. G. Joseph et al., "Coping with the Threat of AIDS: An Approach to Psychosocial Assessment," *American Psychologist,* 39 (November 1984), pp. 1297–1302.

8. J. Bradford, "Reactions of Gay Men to AIDS." Unpublished dissertation, Virginia Commonwealth University, 1986.

9. Joseph et al., "Coping with the Threat of AIDS."
10. Ibid.
11. T. J. Coates, L. Temoshok, and J. Mandel, "Psychosocial Research Is Essential to Understanding and Treating AIDS," *American Psychologist,* 39 (November 1984), p. 1313.
12. L. Altman, "Linking AIDS to Africa Provokes Bitter Debate," *New York Times,* November 21, 1985, pp. 1 and A14.
13. L. Caputo, "Dual Diagnosis: AIDS and Addiction," Briefly Stated section, *Social Work,* 30 (July–August 1985), pp. 361–363.
14. R. Enlow, *Annals of the New York Academy of Science,* November 1985, p. 305.
15. Ibid.
16. Bradford, "Reactions of Gay Men to AIDS"; and Joseph et al., "Coping with the Threat of AIDS."
17. A. Gattozzi, *Psychological and Social Aspects of the Acquired Immune Deficiency Syndrome: Early Findings of Research Supported by the NIMH* (Rockville, Md.: Scientific Communications Branch, National Institute of Mental Health, 1986), p. 17.
18. Dreher, "The Psychosocial Aspects of AIDS."
19. Joseph et al., "Coping with the Threat of AIDS," p. 1302.
20. John L. Martin and Carole S. Vance, "Behavioral and Psychosocial Factors in AIDS: Methodological and Substantive Issues," *American Psychologist,* 39 (November 1984), pp. 1303–1308.
21. Gattozzi, *Psychological and Social Aspects of the Acquired Immune Deficiency Syndrome.*
22. *Cited in* ibid., p. 6.
23. Martin and Vance, "Behavioral and Psychosocial Factors in AIDS."
24. Joseph et al., "Coping with the Threat of AIDS."
25. According to K. Siegel, as cited in Gattozzi, *Psychological and Social Aspects of the Acquired Immune Deficiency Syndrome,* p. 11, the health-belief model "states that a person's willingness to adopt or maintain a preventive health behavior is conditioned upon his belief that, first, the condition to be prevented is serious; second, he perceives himself as personally vulnerable; and, third, he believes that the action he is being asked to adopt will be effective in preventing the disease."
26. L. B. Puchall and P. N. Van Ness, "A Survey of Gay Men's Knowledge and Concern about AIDS: Self-reported Impact on Sexual Practices and Attitudes." Unpublished manuscript, Washington, D.C., 1985.
27. D. G. Ostrow et al., as cited in Gattozzi, *Psychological and Social Aspects of the Acquired Immune Deficiency Syndrome.*
28. Ibid., p. 20.
29. Bradford, "Reactions of Gay Men to AIDS."
30. Dreher, "The Psychosocial Aspects of AIDS."
31. *See* ibid.; S. E. Nichols, Jr., "Psychiatric Aspects of AIDS," *Psychosomatics,* 24 (December 1983), pp. 1083–1089; and E. Kübler-Ross, *On Death and Dying* (New York: Macmillan Co., 1969).

32. *Diagnostic and Statistical Manual of Mental Disorders (Third Edition)* (Washington, D.C.: American Psychiatric Association, 1980); and J. C. B. Holland and S. Tross, as cited in Dreher, "The Psychosocial Aspects of AIDS," p. 17.

33. *See* Gattozzi, *Psychological and Social Aspects of the Acquired Immune Dificiency Syndrome.*

34. *See* Joseph et al., "Coping with the Threat of AIDS."

35. Ibid.

36. Dreher, "The Psychosocial Aspects of AIDS."

37. S. Perry and P. Jacobsen, "Neuropsychiatric Manifestations of AIDS—Spectrum Disorders," *Hospital and Community Psychiatry,* 37 (December 1986), p. 135.

38. Dreher, "The Psychosocial Aspects of AIDS," p. 22.

39. Ibid.

40. Ibid., p. 23.

41. J. Rabin, "AIDS and Gay Bathhouses: A Constitutional Analysis," *Journal of Health Politics, Policy and Law,* 10 (Winter 1986), p. 729.

42. Dreher, "The Psychosocial Aspects of AIDS," p. 10.

4

Meeting the Psychosocial Needs of People with AIDS

Judy Macks

Persons with AIDS face a complex set of psychosocial needs and issues as they confront the impact of the diagnosis on their lives.[1] Various models of psychological responses to the diagnosis of AIDS have been outlined, such as the situational distress model of crisis[2] and adaptive responses by stage and task.[3] Many of the psychological responses to and coping mechanisms for dealing with AIDS are similar to those of other life-threatening illnesses, such as cancer and heart disease.[4] However, the social and political nature of AIDS, as well as the ways in which it is transmitted, set it apart from other diseases. The fact that AIDS invokes cultural taboos about homosexuality, sex, death, and drugs accounts for the stigma attached to the illness. This stigma plays a significant role in the individual's adaption and response to the diagnosis of AIDS. Therefore, any comprehensive biopsychosocial program must address the psychological as well as the sociocultural impact of AIDS on those affected by the disease. This article describes one such program in San Francisco that incorporates a biopsychosocial model and discusses the psychosocial needs of persons with AIDS, the special problems of the diverse populations affected by AIDS, and relevant services, both those that deal with specific psychosocial needs and the range of interventions that may be used for treating other problems. The article concludes with the implications of these needs and problems for improving the delivery of services to persons with AIDS and for developing sound social policies.

San Francisco Program

In 1984, San Francisco General Hospital's AIDS Activities Division and the AIDS Health Project of the University of California, San Francisco (UCSF), jointly designed and implemented a comprehensive program of psychosocial intervention for persons with AIDS and ARC. San Francisco General Hospital provides primary medical care through a multidisciplinary team to persons with AIDS and ARC in its inpatient and outpatient units. The multidisciplinary team coordinates the treatment planning, resources, and services of the inpatient and outpatient units in the hospital in collaboration with community-based services for this population. The psychosocial team at the hospital includes a social worker from the general medical service, a social worker from the UCSF AIDS Health Project, and a peer counselor. The team addresses the concrete needs (benefits, housing, transportation, and so forth), as well as the mental health needs of patients with AIDS and ARC. Psychosocial assessments are obtained for new patients as often as possible; however, because of the volume of clients, baseline data are not available for all patients.

The social worker from the AIDS Health project coordinates the Mental Health Services for Persons with AIDS program at San Francisco General Hospital and offers five services that are designed to meet psychosocial needs: information and referral, psychosocial assessment, crisis intervention, brief therapy, and group interventions. Information and referral services assist clients in obtaining appropriate medical, mental health, social service, and AIDS-specific services, as well as educate clients about the medical aspects of the illness. Psychosocial assessments are completed for clients who receive additional mental health services from the clinic. Crisis intervention services, provided to clients in acute psychological crisis, often require the involvement of the city's community mental health system and the psychiatric consultation services of the hospital. Frequently, clients use brief therapy as an interim service when ongoing psychotherapy services are not immediately available. Group interventions include stress-management groups and couples groups. In the stress management groups, clients learn skills and techniques to manage stress and fluctuating moods and increase social support. The couples groups provide educational support and therapeutic intervention, improve communication between the partners, and enhance individual support systems outside the couple relationship. Both groups are short-term (six to eight weeks) closed groups and are based on a cognitive-behavioral model.

Psychosocial and demographic data were available for 73 of the 301 clients with AIDS or ARC who utilized one or more of these services between March 1984 and November 1985. The all-male sample was primarily gay (91 percent) and white (85 percent); also Latino (7 percent); black (4 percent); and native American (4 percent). The men, whose mean age was 35 years, had lived in the San Francisco Bay Area for a mean of 7.8

years. An equal percentage lived alone (32 percent), with a lover/partner (32 percent), or with roommates (29 percent); the remaining 7 percent did not answer the question. The majority (60 percent) was unemployed and receiving some type of public assistance (78 percent). A highly educated group, nearly half (46 percent) had completed college, and 60 percent had incomes that ranged from $10,000 to $30,000 before their illness. A majority (53 percent) had been in psychotherapy or counseling in their lives, 28 percent had had a problem with alcohol or substance use, and 16 percent had a history of psychiatric hospitalization. Most of the men expressed a desire to make changes in the areas of stress management (89 percent) and coping with depression (83 percent), as well as in diet/nutrition (65 percent), exercise (64 percent), social support (56 percent), coping with recent losses and grief (52 percent), and sexual practices (42 percent).

The next sections describe the psychosocial needs of the populations affected by AIDS, both their special problems and general problems that can be dealt with by a range of interventions. The discussion is based on the author's experiences in the Mental Health Services for People with AIDS program, as well as on her review of the literature.

Special Problems of High-Incidence Groups

All people with AIDS share the profound despair of learning that they have a life-threatening illness, as well as the needs to manage anticipatory grief and crisis periods; the loss of status, control, and social supports; and the stigma associated with AIDS. However, each identified high-incidence group had certain special concerns, to which practitioners and researchers should be sensitive. These special concerns are summarized in this section; the interventions necessary to deal with them and other common psychosocial concerns of people with AIDS are discussed in the next sections.

Services for gay and bisexual men must be sensitive to the cultural, economic, ethnic, political, and social commonalities and diversity of gay communities. Such services must communicate understanding and acceptance in a nonjudgmental atmosphere as well as acknowledge the impact of homophobia, discrimination, and rejection. In addition, practitioners and researchers must confront the significant legal and ethical issues that affect gay men whose civil rights are not protected.

Similarly, practitioners who serve intravenous drug users, both gay and heterosexual, must have knowledge about the use and abuse of drugs and demonstrate sensitivity to the similarities and differences within the racially and sexually diverse populations of drug abusers. Of particular importance is the need for culturally appropriate and relevant services and accessible treatment programs.

Women with AIDS have unique problems as a result of being diagnosed with a disease that is primarily identified as a male disease. Their feelings of isolation, secrecy, and rejection are more acute than that of men with

AIDS because they belong to diverse communities that usually have little access to information about AIDS. In addition, they have special needs as a result of their reproductive capabilities, including concern about transmitting the HIV to their unborn children, decisions about pregnancy, problems involved in caring for their young children with AIDS, and civil liberties issues related to reproductive freedom.

Hemophiliacs with AIDS face the double burden of having two medical illnesses that often result in discrimination and misunderstanding. Many are angry because they think that their exposure to AIDS could have been prevented. Practitioners who serve this group must be aware of both the physical realities of the dual medical diagnoses and the emotional issues faced by hemophiliacs and their families.[5]

Special Needs of Persons with ARC

The lack of a consistent medical definition of ARC points to some of the difficulties that people with ARC face regarding their medical condition. Although they have the same psychosocial problems as do persons with AIDS, they have some unique concerns as well. Most significantly, higher levels of distress, depression, and anxiety, attributed primarily to a higher degree of uncertainty associated with this diagnosis, have been documented among persons with ARC.[6] Because they feel they are living in a state of limbo, persons with ARC may become preoccupied with symptoms, immobilized, and functionally impaired. (Ironically, some persons with ARC feel a sense of relief on receiving a diagnosis of AIDS.) Most people with ARC have limited access to financial, emotional, and social supports, and many, even those with disabling conditions, are not granted presumptive eligibility for benefits for which persons with AIDS are immediately eligible. Finally, many persons with ARC report difficulties in obtaining support from friends and family members, particularly if their symptoms are vague and friends doubt their validity. The entire range of interventions for persons with AIDS, which are described in the next sections, are applicable to persons with ARC, as are the implications for the delivery of services and public policy that are discussed at the end of this article.

Informational Services

People with AIDS must sort through rapidly changing medical and epidemiologic information to make informed choices about their health care. This task can be overwhelming, given the amount of information that is reported regularly in the media and medical journals. That many important medical questions related to treatment, prognosis, and the course of the illness cannot yet be answered engenders confusion and anxiety in many. Therefore, it is essential that mental health and social service professionals, as well as medical professionals, give clients accurate information, whether individually or in groups, to maximize their sense of control over their lives and to minimize the frustrations and uncertainty that they feel.

In particular, clients require information about the medical aspects of AIDS, ongoing treatment options and their side effects, precautions to be taken to control infections, the course of the illness, the transmission of the disease, including guidelines for reducing the risk of transmission. Often, health professionals impart this information at a time of crisis, when clients are unable to retain the information. Therefore, it is important for every practitioner to assess each client's level of knowledge and to educate him or her accordingly.

Clients need access to a wide range of services, including medical, mental health, alternative therapies, and social services. To facilitate the utilization of information and referral services, it is helpful to compile a written list of available resources.

Many clients also need to be made aware of the normative and adaptive emotional responses that they may experience throughout the course of the illness. Knowing what to expect in advance and being reassured that certain responses are normal and common can allay their fears and anxieties about decompensation and the loss of control.

Concrete Services

A person with AIDS may need a range of concrete services, including financial assistance, housing, transportation, home health care, and legal service. It is essential for clients to obtain financial assistance quickly, given the terminal nature of the illness, the rapid progression of the disease, and the continued need for medical services in both inpatient and outpatient settings. Housing concerns may be critical for a person with AIDS who suddenly cannot meet rent or mortgage payments, has been evicted from an apartment because of his or her diagnosis, has moved suddenly to a new area to seek better medical attention, or has a history of unstable living situations before the diagnosis. Women with AIDS who have children have an even more difficult time finding housing that accepts children.

Important and complex legal issues may arise; wills, power of attorney, custody decisions, funeral arrangements, and decisions regarding life supports need to be documented legally. Legal documentation is especially significant for the gay client, who wishes his partner to retain power of attorney and other primary decision-making roles for him. Because the gay relationship is not protected by law, legal documentation protects the client and his partner from intervention by the client's family, which is not legally required to act according to the client's wishes.

Acting in the role of advocates, social workers can provide critical services to persons with AIDS by quickly accessing financial resources and housing, legal, medical, and mental health services. Emergency services, such as housing or presumptive eligibility for Medicaid/Medi-Cal and disability benefits from social security, are not readily available in many areas. Similarly, subsidized independent living situations that offer low-cost housing are scarce. Social workers can be instrumental in developing new programs such as these by advocating, organizing, and planning. They also can play an important role in the complex legal dilemmas that persons with AIDS face by raising the necessary issues, identifying appropriate resources, and facilitating referrals.

Substance Abuse Services

Some people with AIDS are recovering addicts and alcoholics. These individuals often experience profound stress from dealing with AIDS as well as from the recovery from substance abuse and therefore require strong emotional support. Others may need assistance in locating drug treatment programs or in determining the degree to which drugs and alcohol interfere with their lives. Still others have such a severe addiction to drugs that they continue to share needles and hence continue to expose others to the disease. Substance abuse treatment programs, both residential and outpatient, must be both accessible and sensitive to persons with AIDS, especially to women with AIDS who have children or who are pregnant. Furthermore, all professionals and clients in substance abuse programs should be informed about the medical, epidemiologic, psychosocial, and risk-reduction aspects of AIDS.

Services for Neuropsychiatric Complications

The prevalence of neurological complications in clients with AIDS has been documented in the literature.[7] Researchers estimate that 30–75 percent of people with AIDS may experience some degree of cognitive impairment, which can be caused by such opportunistic infections as toxoplasmosis or cryptococcal meningitis or from the infection of the brain with HIV.[8] Clients who experience organically based symptoms, including short-term memory loss, confusion, disorientation, depressive symptoms, or behavioral changes, require intervention and support.

These clients should be referred for medical and psychiatric assessment to ascertain the etiology and potential treatment of the presenting symptoms. Clients and members of their support system, including family members, need to be educated about the cognitive, behavioral, and emotional aspects of dementia, as well as what can be expected both prognostically and on a day-to-day basis. Family members will need both practical assistance in the care of their loved one, as well as instruction in developing interventions to help the person who is confused, disoriented, and experiencing short-term memory loss. For example, large calendars, lists of activities for the day, verbal reminders and cues, and the use of simple language can help the demented client. Family members also may need assistance in assessing the client's intentions and responding to his or her difficult behavior.

Problems that Require a Range of Interventions

This section describes four problems—the management of distressing feelings, the management of crises, the loss of status, and the loss of social support—that can be dealt with by a range of interventions. The psychosocial interventions designed to address these problems are discussed.

Management of Distressing Feelings

Many clients with AIDS request assistance in dealing with their distressing feelings, which they describe as a roller coaster of emotions—mood fluctuations compounded by an overwhelming sense of hopelessness and helplessness. Persons with AIDS go through an anticipatory grief process that is similar to the process experienced by cancer patients. The stages of this process, which were identified by Kübler-Ross, include denial, anger, bargaining, depression, and acceptance.[9]

Clients with AIDS experience multiple losses as well, including changes in sexual behavior and intimate relationships, disfigurement and an impaired self-image, changes in employment patterns, and the loss of previous sources of self-esteem. Furthermore, many are grieving for a partner, friends, or acquaintances who already have died from AIDS.

Sociocultural factors and societal responses to AIDS seem to exacerbate the distressing reactions of guilt, self-blame, and lowered self-esteem. These feelings may stem from unresolved conflicts about one's sexual orientation or internalized manifestations of homophobia, racism, or sexism. Messages commonly expressed in the media that blame homosexuals or prostitutes for this disease significantly influence an individual's feelings about the illness. Rather than identifying the cause of the illness as a virus, many feel they have caused the disease because of who they are or how they have lived.

Some individuals experience feelings of contamination, particularly in association with sexuality and physical-affectional closeness. Although these feelings are common for people who face any life-threatening illness, they may be exacerbated in persons with AIDS because of the sexual transmissibility of the disease. These feelings can be intensified further by the unnecessary and irrational procedures adopted by some providers and institutions, such as excessive use of masks, gowns, gloves, and goggles in situations that do not require such precautions.

Actual or feared rejection also contributes to high levels of distress. Many persons with AIDS experience rejection by their families, partners, social support systems, and employers. Whether real or anticipated, this rejection can profoundly effect their psychosocial functioning.

What often underlies many distressing feelings is the desire to discover an internal sense of hope and empowerment that can help one focus on living, rather than dying. The development or maintenance of adaptive coping skills, such as denial, repression or sublimation, an increase in the sense of the mastery of and control over one's life, the maximization of one's decision-making power, involvement in Western medicine or alternative healing therapies, and involvement in productive activities, can contribute to a hopeful and positive attitude. However, since many of these coping skills can become destructive or maladaptive, practitioners need to be aware of countertransference issues and be willing to confront clients who exhibit this self-destructive behavior.

Management of Crises

A number of periods of crisis occur during the progression of this disease. Such crises include the time of the initial diagnosis, the onset or recurrence of a particular symptom or infection, a sudden or profound loss of mobility, the failure of treatment, rejection by a family member, or the terminal stage of the illness. At these times, clients may be prone to psychological decompensation. The premorbid personality, functioning, and coping skills may be the best indicators of their ability to manage these crises.

Persons with AIDS commonly express suicidal ideation at times of crisis, primarily in an attempt to manage feelings of despair, loss of control, helplessness, and the fear of future events. Those who are actively suicidal often have had a clinical history of depression, anxiety, suicide attempts, substance abuse, or character disorder. However, others consider suicide during the final stage of the illness as a means of freeing themselves from further suffering.

Loss of Status

People with AIDS frequently need assistance in adapting psychologically to the many physiological and psychosocial changes that occur throughout the course of the disease that result in their sense of a loss of status. Close to 70 percent of all persons with AIDS are 20–39 years old and often at the beginning or peak of their career. Some may be forced to abandon their source of income, social support, and self-esteem. For others, feelings of failure accompany their disappointment at the realization that their dreams and plans for the future and their intentions of creating a more stable life will never be realized. Interrupted occupational or social functioning, as well as a growing reliance on others for basic care, can lead to a sense of decreased status. The drastic alterations in lifestyle necessitated by chronic fatigue, debilitation, the loss of mobility, and the loss of bodily functions can result in isolation, boredom, the increased use of drugs and alcohol, and depression. As the client increasingly needs to rely on friends, family, and support systems for basic care, loss of independent functioning contributes to the perceived loss of status.

Social Support

The literature documents the ameliorative effects of social supports on depression and the ability to cope with medical illness.[10] The need for adequate social support systems is of primary importance for persons with AIDS.

A diagnosis of AIDS can have a profound impact on the client's social support system. For example, a gay man may be faced with the simultaneous disclosure to his parents that he has been diagnosed with a life-threatening illness and that he is gay. This disclosure is likely to precipitate a crisis for him and his family and can result either in a deleterious or positive outcome. Different but equally disturbing situations may arise for persons in other high-incidence groups.

The emotional responses of the partners or spouses of persons with AIDS are similar to those of the family members of other groups of patients. However, because AIDS is transmitted sexually, these persons have unique concerns as well. Most likely, the partner or spouse has been exposed and possibly infected with HIV through sexual contact with the client who has AIDS. Therefore, the couple must deal with the impact of AIDS on their relationship as well as the uncertainty of the partner's or spouse's future health. The person with AIDS may feel guilty for infecting his partner or spouse. Such concerns add new levels of stress to an already stressful situation.

Psychosocial Interventions

Biopsychosocial Assessment

With a life-threatening disease involving progressive physiological and often cognitive deterioration, a biopsychosocial assessment provides particularly useful information if it is made during the baseline period. The interrelationship of the physiological, psychological, and sociocultural aspects of AIDS for each client must be attended to simultaneously. It becomes particularly important to gather data regarding the person's premorbid personality, coping skills, strengths and weaknesses, risk of psychological decompensation as evidenced by a history of psychiatric problems, occupational and social functioning, family history, use of substances, self-esteem and feelings about AIDS, and particular risk factors. Attention to cultural, religious, and spiritual values and attitudes is critical, especially their relation to communication styles, homosexuality, the use of drugs, and death, dying, and grief.

Crisis Intervention

Many clients require intervention during acute crises. Interventions should be designed to enhance their adaptive and integrative functioning through past and newly acquired coping skills. It is preferable to offer crisis services in medical or community settings because these settings can provide early intervention services and possibly prevent further crises.

Individual Therapy

A wide range of individual interventions—including supportive, cognitive-behavioral, and insight-oriented therapy—can be helpful for the person with AIDS. Individual therapy can be particularly useful in addressing the client's ability to manage distressing feelings and crises, deal with the ramifications of his or her perceived loss of status, enhance support systems, maintain hopefulness, and maximize decision-making skills. It often provides a structure in which to work thorough the stages of anticipatory grief. For some clients, individual therapy may be the intervention of choice. For the chronically mentally disabled, it may be the primary modality in which education and support can be provided effectively.

Groups

Group interventions have been documented to be useful for persons facing life-threatening illnesses.[11] In particular, groups allow for the enhancement of social support by providing clients with the opportunity to discuss issues and problems related to the illness with others who are experiencing similar problems. A range of group modalities has been found to be useful for persons with AIDS, including cognitive-behavioral groups, therapy groups, self-help groups, and groups for family members. For many persons with AIDS, group interventions are sufficient; for others, groups are useful in conjunction with individual treatment. Clients are encouraged or required to be in individual therapy while participating in a group if they are assessed to be at a high risk for psychological decompensation, have a characterological disorder, or are actively suicidal. Some clients are screened from groups if, at the time of assessment, it seems that they would be too disruptive to the group or would be unable to gain from the group experience.

The short-term closed-group model has both advantages and disadvantages over other models of group intervention. For persons facing a life-threatening illness, a short-term closed-group model can provide consistency, thereby enhancing the development of social support. The structure provides a container for overwhelming feelings and a context for developing a sense of empowerment and hope about continuing to live as fully as possible. This model also provides the best opportunity for maintaining the integrity of a group, given the fluctuation in physical status and the high mortality rate of people with AIDS. Although long-term groups offer the opportunity for in-depth therapeutic intervention, they are difficult in this situation because of the increasing debilitation and frequent deaths of group members. The major disadvantage to closed-group models is the significant lag time that may occur between the client's initial contact with the group facilitator or agency and the beginning of the group. For those who require immediate intervention or whose emotional or physical state may prevent them from making a commitment to a time-limited or ongoing closed group, drop-in groups can be especially useful.

Implications for the Delivery of Services

The AIDS epidemic undoubtedly requires a multidisciplinary approach to the care of clients with AIDS and regular collaboration among medical, mental health, social service, substance abuse, and community organization professionals, as well as community activists. Clearly, no single service or intervention can meet the complex biopsychosocial needs of persons with AIDS.

During the first five years of the AIDS epidemic, services were designed and implemented in reaction to the immediate crisis. Now that it is known that this epidemic will be with us for some time and become more widespread, it is essential to assess the needs of the various populations involved and to evaluate current programs to develop a long-range plan for comprehensive systems to deliver services at the local, state, and federal levels.

Models of care will differ geographically because they will reflect the social, economic, and political characteristics of the communities that are most affected by AIDS, the local community at large, and the organization and structure of the local health care system.[12] However, an effective approach in any community will link hospital-based services with public health, mental health, and substance abuse systems; private practitioners, community-based groups, AIDS agencies, volunteers, and representatives of the populations that are most heavily affected by AIDS.

The availability of outpatient services is of particular importance in terms of the quality and cost effectiveness of the care that is provided.[13] Services that allow for decreased hospital stays and adequate home care include practical support, comprehensive home health care and hospices, housing and other residential facilities, foster care, psychosocial support, and mental health crisis services. Input from the populations that are most at risk of contracting AIDS will be an important clue to the development of appropriate and effective models of care.

Providers of health, mental health, and social services need comprehensive training and education programs about AIDS. Such programs should cover the medical, epidemiologic, psychosocial, and neuropsychiatric aspects of AIDS, as well as provide an opportunity to discuss emotional reactions to working with these clients. In addition, attention must be paid to the development of sensitivity to the particular needs of persons in high-incidence groups.

Many professionals express concern about the problems of working with persons with AIDS because of the intense physical and emotional demands on staff members. Administrators must address the concerns of staff members if they are to provide high-quality care for the clients as well as to prevent burnout in staff members. Various forms of staff support can be developed and integrated into a variety of work settings. Staff groups, particularly for those who work directly with persons with AIDS, have found sessions that are facilitated by professionals to be useful.

Implications for Public Policy

Public policy must address the AIDS epidemic as a public health crisis from the perspective of prevention, treatment, research, the delivery of services, funding, and the impact of AIDS on the health care delivery system. Prevention must be addressed nationally in a reasonable and responsible fashion. AIDS is a preventable disease for those who have not yet been infected with HIV. The only reasonable approach, in lieu of a cure or vaccine, is a massive program of public health education that reaches all people and is simple in presentation, culturally sensitive, and multilingual.

Funding for AIDS research must be a priority. Funds also must be allocated for the development of comprehensive health care delivery systems that meet the complex needs of persons with AIDS at the local, state, and federal levels. The development of such systems can be accomplished by augmenting the funding of existing health care delivery systems that may be working at maximum capacity and by continuing to fund existing and new AIDS agencies.

Economic analyses have documented the cost effectiveness of outpatient and home care services.[14] A comparative analysis of the length and cost of hospital stays for AIDS patients in New York City and San Francisco found that the average length of a hospital stay is 11.7 days in San Francisco and 25.4 days in New York City, and that the average cost of a hospital stay per patient is therefore significantly lower in San Francisco ($9,044) than in New York City ($20,320).[15] This difference has been attributed, in large part, to the availability in San Francisco of an array of outpatient services that meet the basic home health care and psychosocial needs of persons with AIDS. The appropriation of adequate funds for residential programs—independent living situations and long-term nursing care facilities—as an alternative to hospitals, as well as home health care services and hospice programs, will prove to both cost effective and more efficient in meeting the needs of persons with AIDS.

Public policy must address the long-range implications of AIDS as a spectrum disorder. A comprehensive array of services must be available to persons diagnosed with ARC or HIV (infection or seropositivity). Health care systems will be significantly affected by the increased incidence of long-term disablities and AIDS-related dementia in these populations.

In sum, local inpatient, outpatient, and community-based services for persons with AIDS must be coordinated if an effective integrated system of delivering health care services is to be developed and maintained. With adequate funding from local, state, and federal governments, the complex biopsychosocial needs of persons with AIDS can be met in a humane and cost-effective manner.

Notes and References

1. D. L. Wolcott, F. I. Fawzy, and R. O. Pasnau, "Acquired Immune Deficiency Syndrome (AIDS) and Consultation–Liaison Psychiatry," *General Hospital Psychiatry,* 7 (1985), pp. 280–292; G. Christ, L. Wiener, and R. Moynihan, "Psychosocial Issues in AIDS," *Psychiatric Annals,* 16 (1986), pp. 173–179; K. Siegel, "AIDS: The Social Dimension," *Psychiatric Annals,* 16 (1986), pp. 168–172; M. Cohen and H. Weisman, "A Biopsychosocial Approach to AIDS," *Psychosomatics,* 27 (1986), pp. 245–249; D. J. Lopez and G. S. Getzel, "Helping Gay Aids Patients in Crisis," *Social Casework,* 65 (September 1984), pp. 387–394; J. S. Mandel, *"The Psychosocial Challenge of AIDS and ARC," Focus,* 2 (January 1986), pp. 1–2; and J. W. Dilley et al., "Findings in Psychiatric Consultations with Patients with Acquired Immune Deficiency Syndrome," *American Journal of Psychiatry,* 142 (1985), p. 1.

2. S. E. Nichols, "Psychosocial Reactions of Persons with Acquired Immunodeficiency Syndrome," *Annals of Internal Medicine,* 103 (1985), pp. 765–769.

3. J. W. Dilley, "Treatment Interventions and Approaches to Care of Patients with Acquired Immune Deficiency Syndrome," in S. E. Nichols and D. G. Astrow, eds., *Psychiatric Implications of Acquired Immune Deficiency Syndrome* (Washington, D.C.: American Psychiatric Press, 1984), pp. 62–70.

4. Wolcott, Fawzy, and Pasnau: "Acquired Immune Deficiency Syndrome (AIDS) and Consultation–Liaison Psychiatry"; M. Forstein, "The Psychosocial Impact of the Acquired Immunodeficiency Syndrome," *Seminars in Oncology,* 11 (1984), pp. 77–82; S. Morin, K. Charles, and A. Mahyon, "The Psychological Impact of AIDS on Gay Men," *American Psychologist,* 39 (1984), pp. 1288–1293; and S. Nichols, "Psychiatric Aspects of AIDS," *Psychosomatics,* 24 (1983), pp. 1083–1089.

5. M. Helquist, "Hemophilia and AIDS," *Focus,* 6 (May 1986), p. 3.

6. Mandel, "The Psychosocial Challenge of AIDS and ARC."

7. Wolcott, Fawzy, and Pasnau, "Acquired Immune Deficiency Syndrome (AIDS) and Consultation–Liaison Psychiatry"; R. J. Loewenstein and S. S. Shartstein, "Neuropsychiatric Aspects of Acquired Immune Deficiency Syndrome," *International Journal of Psychiatry in Medicine,* 13 (1983–1984), pp. 255–260; B. G. Gazzard et al., "Clinical Findings and Serological Evidence of HTLV III Infection in Homosexual Contacts of Patients with AIDS and Persistent Generalized Lymphadenopathy in London," *Lancet* (1984), pp. 480–485; and J. Holland and S. Tross, "The Psychosocial and Neuropsychiatric

Sequelae of the Acquired Immunodeficiency Syndrome and Related Disorders," *Annals of Internal Medicine,* 103 (1985), pp. 760–764.

8. W. D. Snider et al., "Neurological Complications of Acquired Immune Deficiency Syndrome: Analysis of 50 Patients," *Annals of Neurology,* 14 (1983), pp. 403–418; D. E. Bresden and R. Messing, "Neurological Syndromes Heralding the Acquired Immune Deficiency Syndrome" (abstract), *Annals of Neurology,* 14 (1983), p. 141; and S. Perry and S. Tross, "Psychiatric Problems of AIDS Inpatients at the New York Hospital: Preliminary Report," *Public Health Reports,* 99 (1984), pp. 200–205.

9. E. Kübler-Ross, *On Death and Dying* (New York: Macmillan Co., 1969).

10. S. Cavanaugh, D. Clark, and R. Gibbons, "Diagnosing Depression in the Hospitalized Medically Ill," *Psychosomatics,* 24 (1983), pp. 809–815; R. Moos, ed., *Coping With Physical Illness* (New York: Plenum Medical Book Co., 1977); and S. Cobb, "Social Support as a Moderator of Life Stress," *Psychomatic Medicine,* 38 (1976), pp. 300–314.

11. R. H. Rahe, H. W. Ward, and V. Hayes, "Brief Group Therapy in Myocardial Infarction Rehabilitation: Three to Four Year Follow-up of a Controlled Trial," *Psychosomatic Medicine,* 41 (1979), pp. 229–242; T. P. Hacket, "The Use of Groups in the Rehabilitation of the Post-coronary Patient," *Advances in Cardiology,* 24 (1978), pp. 127–135; and D. Spiegel and I. D. Yalom, "A Support Group for Dying Patient," *International Journal of Group Psychotherapy,* 28 (1978), pp. 233–235.

12. P. S. Arno and R. G. Hughes, "Local Policy Response to the AIDS Epidemic: New York and San Francisco." Unpublished paper, Institute for Health Policy Studies, University of California, San Francisco, June 1986.

13. P. S. Arno, "The Nonprofit Sector's Response to the AIDS Epidemic: Community-based Services in San Francisco." Unpublished paper, Institute for Health Policy Studies, University of California, San Francisco, February 1986.

14. Arno and Hughes, "Local Policy Response to the AIDS Epidemic: New York and San Francisco."

15. D. J. Sencer and V. E. Botnick, *"Report to the Mayor: New York City's Response to the AIDS Crisis"* (New York: Office of the Mayor, December 1985).

5

The Family and AIDS

Deborah A. Newmark and Edward H. Taylor

AIDS, like all illnesses, affects the entire family system. However, no other modern disease or social crisis except AIDS has created the need for redefining the composition of the family, safeguarding the civil liberties of family members, and ensuring minimal community services for families in which a member has AIDS. Beyond regular mourning and the usual difficulties associated with catastrophic illness, family members must contend with unusual and complex family systems that inhibit communication and problem-solving. Each member has real and imagined problems, such as isolation, fears of transmissibility, stigma, and confrontation with homosexuality or drug abuse in the family unit. Each individual, like the person with AIDS, often feels attacked by and separated from the other family members as well as the community at large.

These difficulties do not end after normal grieving but are reenacted when family members reach new developmental stages, encounter limited community resources, and concern themselves with their physical well-being. The author's observations drawn from clinical practice suggest that emotional, developmental, and concrete problems are compounded by the lack of community support services to the complete family. Their extensive interviews with patients, traditional family members, and significant others have produced evidence that new family structures and subsystems must be conceptualized if social workers and other helping professionals are to intervene successfully with the families of persons with AIDS.

New Family Systems

The population of persons with AIDS includes, among others, individuals who live in familial structures that parallel the traditional nuclear family in many ways but that retain distinctive characteristics, including the lack of legal sanction, that significantly influence the quality of life of their members. The homosexual couple unit, for example, is not protected by law or recognized as legitimate by society. Because it is not accepted, its members may suffer economic, social, and professional disadvantages.

Most of the clients who receive social work services at the National Institutes of Health are men, ranging in age from 20–49 years. In addition to those who live in homosexual couple units, these men live in the following types of families: (1) the family of origin, consisting of the parents and their adult children; (2) the nuclear family, which includes a husband and wife, with or without offspring; (3) a bisexual marital arrangement involving a husband and wife, with or without offspring, and the husband's gay lover; and (4) an unmarried heterosexual couple unit.

These family systems reflect the new values and mores that evolved in relation to the high rate of divorce and the gay rights movement. The units are fluid and may change over time. In addition to these family systems, there are those homosexual units in which the partner with AIDS receives emotional support not only from his gay partner but from his former wife and children. The spouse and children from the previous marriage represent the traditional life that the person with AIDS experienced before he came out publicly as a homosexual.

These complex family subsystems have the potential of creating what Bronfenbrenner called "exosystems," and becoming sources of conflict.[1] An exosystem is any individual or environment that affects another person without the person's knowledge of the exosystem's activity. The person with AIDS may have established complete detached family subsystems, isolated from other family members, that become exosystems in relation to the other subsystems. These unknown forces may cause boundary disputes and changes in the family's equilibrium. Individual members may experience a new sense of isolation and detachment as their primary support system shifts and new exosystems are created. Because boundaries and loosely connected subsystems may change quickly, assessments of a family's structure must be frequently updated.

Major Problems

Families must deal with a number of problems that arise when a member is diagnosed as having AIDS. The major problems, which are discussed in this section, are isolation, the fear of contagion, stigmatization, and confronting homosexuality.

Isolation

It is important to recognize that each family member confronts social isolation from the established family unit, the neighborhood, the larger community, and the macro political system. During the course of clinical interventions, many families have identified isolation as one of their most difficult social and psychological problems. They often report that the following factors exacerbate their sense of detachment and isolating behaviors: (1) the emotional pain of dealing with a life-threatening illness of such magnitude; (2) the fear of contagion, which requires taking precautions and necessitates some physical separation from the person with AIDS; (3) stigmatization, which necessitates secrecy from customary support systems; and (4) controversy among the family systems.

Isolation within Isolation. Isolation within isolation occurs when heterosexual family members do not include or accept the afflicted person's gay friends and lover. Without open communication between traditional and alternative family subsystems, the process by which the entire family system makes decisions becomes dysfunctional. Religious, cultural, and generational differences have a serious impact on such significant decisions as cremation versus burial and euthanasia versus the use of life-sustaining procedures. This type of isolation can be painful to the afflicted person and to his friends and lover. It also prevents family members from having positive relationships with and help from these persons.

Isolation within isolation also arises when individual family members, including the afflicted member, become secretive because they are privy to certain pieces of information that they do not want to share with other family members. This behavior often results in miscommunications that lead to family conflicts. The following is not an unusual scenario:

> Mrs. G, who had been married to Mr. G for 30 years, wondered aloud how he might have contracted AIDS. Because she did not know of his homosexual activity, she postulated that he had contracted the disease through casual contact; therefore, she reasoned that she and their grandchildren were also vulnerable to contagion from such contact. Was it only a matter of time until she too was diagnosed with the illness? Should she prevent her husband from kissing and hugging the grandchildren?

Parents may be kept in the dark about the family member's homosexuality and perhaps about the diagnosis of AIDS as well, being told instead that their son or husband has a rare form of cancer. Because they may learn of the diagnosis in the end stages of the disease, they may feel deprived of part of the mourning process as well as despondent at losing their loved one.

Fear of Transmission

One way the virus, identified as the causative agent, may be transmitted is through sexual contact. Therefore, to avoid contracting AIDS, the spouse or partner usually refrains from sexual relations with the afflicted person. Doing so, however, reinforces his or her feeling of isolation. Some partners or spouses continue to have sexual relations with persons with AIDS, despite this risk, because they do not want to lose the valuable outlet for intimacy that is now time limited.

The difficulty of living with the uncertainty that one might have AIDS causes many partners or spouses to be screened for the virus.[2] When the test result is positive, the individual then must face the ambiguity of not knowing if he or she is to develop a full-blown case of AIDS. The following vignette describes this conflict:

Mrs. B, the widow of a former patient with AIDS-related complex, tested positive for HTLV-III. In addition to her grief, she had to live with the dilemma of not knowing if she would contract the disease. Every time she got a head cold or a sore throat, she wondered if it might be the first sign of AIDS.

The person whose test is positive (the "seropositive person") needs to decide whether to inform a future sexual partner of his or her risk. Persons in this category of seropositivity may feel morally and legally obligated to reveal their condition yet afraid to do so because they might be rejected by a potential partner.

A seropositive woman must make a similar decision about having children. Although she may want to have a child, she probably has been advised by her physician not to become pregnant because she could transmit the virus to the fetus. Furthermore, she does not know whether this warning about not becoming pregnant is temporary or whether she will never be free of the risk throughout her reproductive lifetime.

The person who is responsible for transmitting AIDS may feel guilty for doing so, particularly if he or she has been sexually active outside the relationship and the partner or spouse has been monogamous. Frequent sexual contacts outside the relationship increase the chance of contracting or transmitting AIDS. The following two comments are typical reactions:

Joe (the partner with AIDS) was monogamous with me. I was the one who was sleeping around, and now I've got to live with the fact that I've given him AIDS and I'm off scot-free.

Both Cynthia and I accepted my bisexuality as part of our marriage. But I never thought I'd infect her with AIDS. Now I have to live with the horror of it on a daily basis.

Future predictions indicate that the virus will spread into the heterosexual community and thus have a significant impact on traditional family systems. Individuals who are not monogamous and who have sexual relations with persons whose risk is unknown may become infected, as may those who have sexual intercourse with prostitutes, users of intravenous drugs, or those who received blood transfusions before the development of the HTLV-III antibody test.

Unlike sexual activity, casual contact is not considered to be a factor in the transmission of AIDS. One recent family study indicated that "household contacts who are not sexual partners of, or born to, patients with AIDS are at minimal or no risk of infection with HTLV-III/LAV."[3] However, many family members continue to struggle with their fears of casual contact. Education and reassurance do not always resolve their anxiety. One partner of a man with AIDS reported that his housecleaning activities had escalated to the extent that he was adding ammonia to the dishwashing detergent. The sister of a man with AIDS talked of her fears of driving with him in a car with the windows closed because the air would be stagnant. Despite knowing how the disease is transmitted, she still feared that the virus might be airborne.

Stigma

The society associates AIDS with deviant behavior and holds homosexuals responsible for the epidemic because the disease has primarily afflicted homosexuals.

Because this stigma is so severe, it alienates persons with AIDS and their families from community supports when they are particularly vulnerable. Spouses of persons with AIDS report that they are unable to talk at work about their husbands' illness for fear of losing their jobs. Children and their parents explain that they cannot tell their teachers the reasons for the father's ailing health because they are afraid that the children will be ousted from school. Furthermore, they feel constrained to discuss the disease with friends, neighbors, or colleagues.

The gay partners of persons with AIDS carry the stigma associated with what many have defined as a homosexual disease and the considerable discrimination and social ostracism directed toward the gay community. Furthermore, they are the objects of the homophobia of their partners' families as well as the larger community. The following care may serve as an example:

> Richard was grieving for his partner who had just died from AIDS. He was particularly upset because the obituary read "no survivors." In terms of the family of origin, this information was accurate. However, Richard considered himself to be the deceased person's family—his "lifetime partner"—and consequently felt nonexistent because of his omission from the obituary.

Confronting Homosexuality in the Family

Many parents first learn of their sons' homosexuality when their sons contract AIDS—a realization that is complicated by the fact that their sons are dying. The parents often feel conflict or disappointment because their sons have failed to follow family norms. These norms include the responsibility to procreate and carry on the family name and the implicit duty to take care of one's parents during their declining years. Sometimes disappointment is expressed in an angry manner, as was done by one father who told his son that he had brought the disease on himself. Some parents may deny that their sons are terminally ill, maintaining instead the magical belief that if their sons will give up their gay lifestyles and come home, they will recover. For example, when the parents of a man with AIDS can from rural Alabama to visit their ailing son, they brought "holy oil" from their church and rubbed his body with it in an attempt to heal him. They pleaded with him to come home and recuperate.

Many parents feel responsible for their sons' choice of sexual orientation. In an AIDS support groups, one mother expressed her guilt over her son's homosexuality as if she perceived his behavior to be an indication of her failings as a parent. She spoke of her ignorance of her son's struggle with this problem and lamented her lack of intervention to prevent his homosexual identity from emerging. "If I'd only known of this struggle during his early teenage years when he was probably first conscious of his homosexuality," she said, "then I might have prevented it from happening."

How do social workers help the families of persons with AIDS deal with the problems just described? The next sections discuss the tasks involved in case management and a model for family treatment.

Case Management

When a family member develops a catastrophic illness such as AIDS, the family often needs to become involved with numerous agencies that offer concrete and emotional support services. However, many agencies that provide specialized services have had little or no experience with persons with AIDS and their families. This situation may be confusing, frustrating, and disruptive to health care providers because of the new family system. Therefore, skillful case management, which incorporates the coordination of resources, training in-service skills, psychosocial education, mediation, and advocacy will be necessary to help the family reach and make use of services.

Agencies require education and assistance from the case manager because AIDS triggers highly charged emotional responses in agency workers. Before engaging the family, workers need technical information about the disease, an outlet for ventilation of their anxieties, and advice about intervention. Agency workers are better able to serve the family sensitively and effectively after they explore and express their knowledge of and fears about AIDS.

Furthermore, some workers may welcome the opportunity to rehearse assessment methods and interviewing techniques with the case manager before intervening with the family.[4] Agencies may be advised to use the case manager for individual consultation and leadership in problem-solving conferences. For example, assistance may be needed to reduce real and imagined interagency difficulties caused by including AIDS patients in the organization's service delivery system. The necessity for conducting treatment interventions with community service agencies markedly differentiates the case management of persons with AIDS and their families from the case management of other types of clients because the social worker must simultaneously treat the family and the service providers.

A major case management task is to prepare families to meet with community agencies. Like individuals facing other crises, the families of persons with AIDS must learn to accept help, understand the limitations of the services, and provide the documentation required for establishing eligibility for assistance. However, unlike clients undergoing many other types of crises, families of persons with AIDS must often face the resistance and fear of service providers as well as limited resources. As a result, the system reinforces isolating behaviors and contributes to the psychological pain experienced by the clients.

Moreover, heterosexual family members may be forced for the first time to receive concrete services, education, and support from organizations in the gay community. However, they will not gain the maximum benefits from gay counselors and agencies without substantial preparation that includes the exploration of feelings and values and the clarification of the need for and goals of these services. This problem may be critical for members of a traditional family who were not aware of their son's or spouse's lifestyle before the diagnosis of AIDS or for the family whose loved one is not homosexual. Many of these individuals have had little or no interactions with the gay community and often hold stereotyped perceptions of the lifestyles of gay people.

A Model of Family Treatment

This section describes the components of a model for treating families of persons with AIDS. It includes a discussion of the framework of the model and the importance of group therapy, support groups, and individual therapy.

Framework

Cognitive and existential therapies are the framework for family treatment. These therapies incorporate the following objectives: (1) to identify the thought processes of family members; (2) to focus on the immediate crisis and environmental situation; (3) to label rational, healthy thoughts and to reframe destructive ones; (4) to establish the hope of overcoming negative feelings by reminding the family of past conflicts and disappointments that have been diffused or overcome; (5) to initiate the grief process by clearly stating that the individual is going to die; (6) to utilize the family group process to establish goals for taking care of each other and achieving the highest quality of life that is possible; and (7) to assist the family to discover the existential meaning of the crisis and impending death.[5] The following is an example of statements that a social worker can make to a parent who is confronting his or her son's homosexuality in the early stages of the illness:

■ It is okay to be angry and disappointed that he is not following the family's norms. However, sexual identity is only part of his life.

■ There have been other things in his life that have disappointed you but you resolved them without ending the relationship. Your disappointment about his homosexuality may be softened with time.

■ His life is threatened and this angers you more than his homosexuality. Homosexuality is one small part of the person you know and love, who is about to be taken from you.

■ Your loved one is dying and you feel upset, angry, and helpless.

■ He is not homosexual or dying because you are a bad person or parent [spouse].

■ Your primary duty is to ensure that your son and your family receive the best medical and community assistance that is available.

■ By working together, we will grow, learn, and eventually make sense of this tragedy.

The social worker may change statements such as these to meet the specific needs, ages, and cultural requirements of the family members.

The isolation experienced by the family needs to be acknowledged early in the illness. Because the community's resistance and the fear of being alone without help are real issues, social work must include active advocacy, behavioral modeling, legal representations, and therapy with the family and social support networks. Many families will need to be taught how to be assertive with agency representatives, peers, and members of the extended family through a combination of assertiveness training and demonstrations of social work advocacy techniques.[6] Accompanying the family on visits to hospitals, schools, community agencies, places of worship, and their jobs may reassure them, educate others, and provide opportunities for advocacy and the reinforcement of appropriate types of assertiveness.

Home visits by the social worker support the family, help resolve transportation difficulties, and serve as a model for neighbors, relatives, and community workers. Frequent home visits demonstrate that the virus is not contracted through ordinary contact with the afflicted person or his home environment.

Whenever possible, the social worker should assess the potential for support by friends, neighbors, relatives, and co-workers of the person with AIDS and of other members of the immediate family. He or she should compile a list of these members of the support network and call on them as needed. The social worker can attempt to allay these persons' fears by providing information and support, first through telephone calls, letters, and visits without the family and then through arranging short visits with selected family members who do not have AIDS. The tone of these visits should be informal and friendly, and their location should be a neutral, non-threatening one. These visits will not be therapeutic for the family, however, until each support person understands the disease process and the psychological pain experienced by the family.

Once the support persons learn to control their anxiety and behavior, they and the family can make arrangements for transportation, child care, weekly visits, and so forth. Interventions of this type are successful only if accurate assessments have been made of the family and the support network. The worker also must have a basic understanding of cognitive, behavioral, and family network therapies.

To deal effectively with familial and community problems, the person with AIDS, his or her partner, and the family members need ongoing legal advice and representation. Family members may find it difficult to advocate for themselves and the patient without a sound understanding of local, state, and federal public health, employment, and civil rights laws.[7] For one example, what legal rights does an individual have if access to or membership in a private or public organization is restricted because the person has been in contact with the AIDS virus? For another example, family members need to be advised of any legal responsibilities, liabilities, or possible legal actions that could result directly or indirectly from the illness. Members of the new or nontraditional family cannot function assertively without having a clear understanding of their legal rights and responsibilities and the benefits to which they are entitled.

During the early stages of the illness, they should address with a lawyer such issues as the drawing up or changing of wills, estate planning, the review of insurance policies and potential options, and establishing a power of attorney. These actions have two serious psychological implications; they acknowledge that the ill person is going to die and that the control of important aspects of the person's life will soon pass to another. For some family members a team approach, which includes the contributions of a social worker, a lawyer, and a member of the clergy, may be necessary.

Group Therapy and Support Groups

In a study for the National Institutes of Health, Newmark found that professionally facilitated support groups that are initiated early in the disease process significantly modify the participants' feelings of loneliness and alienation.[8] The objectives of such groups are as follows: (1) to facilitate communication, (2) to encourage sharing, (3) to provide information about the disease, (4) to alleviate anxiety, and (5) to foster the idea that this is a mutual experience.[9] Support groups may be composed of one category of person, such as widows, parents, or lovers whereas therapy groups usually are organized along the lines of diagnostic and developmental issues. Support groups are generally open ended and loosely structured than are therapy groups, which are more clearly defined and leader dependent. Furthermore, support groups encourage ongoing communication and networking. The objectives of support groups are focused on daily and immediate needs, whereas therapy groups often focus on developmental issues and long-term goals. Both types of interventions are useful and may be helpful at different phases of the crisis.

In groups, it is important that certain populations should not be mixed. For example, do not mix those who are learning about AIDS and whose loved one is still alive with those who have lost a loved one. Those who are in the process of accepting the disease and its consequences may be using such defense mechanisms as denial and sublimation that may be necessary for them to cope. Therefore, it may be antitherapeutic to expose them to people who are further along in the grief process.

Individual Therapy

In addition to family and group interventions, individual therapy is recommended for spouses, partners, and children. In individual therapy, the social worker can provide the client with immediate crisis intervention by facilitating communication, encouraging the ventilation of feelings, and mitigating anxiety during frequent in-person sessions and telephone consultations. The long-range objective of such therapy is to explore continuing developmental issues that are related to the trauma created by AIDS.

The partner, whether defined by traditional or alternative lifestyles, needs a stable therapeutic relationship to help him or her come to terms with the loss or impending loss of the primary love object, assume new roles, be strong emotionally, and cope with the possibility of having contracted AIDS.

Children must readdress the loss and discover new insight into feelings and information about AIDS at successive developmental stages. Young children may be helped to express their feelings and to sort out their confusion over the meaning of separation and death through drawing and play therapy. As they grow older, children must integrate increasingly difficult perceptions, which often are in conflict with social norms, of their fathers' history, illness, and death.

Conclusion

The magnitude of the AIDS crisis partially may be understood by considering the mobility of the U.S. population and current sexual norms, which contribute to the spread of AIDS, as well as the number of family members who are associated with each afflicted person. While medical researchers search for effective treatments, screening tools, and a vaccine, social workers must address the psychosocial needs of the family and the afflicted person and advocate for the rights of persons with AIDS to receive health insurance and emergency, acute, and chronic care from public and private health care facilities.

Most local agencies need to train their staffs before planning multidimensional services for families of persons with AIDS because social workers will not be able to adapt their generic social work skills to specific interventions without understanding the medical, psychological, and social implications of the illness. The agencies must have access to empirical data that are sensitive to the cultures of the various populations that are at risk of contracting AIDS before they can define, no less provide, assistance, support, education, and psychotherapy that are based on culturally relevant methods, rather than on global generalities.

Although AIDS is a national problem, it is experienced by the family as a personal crisis. Therefore, agencies should establish multitrack service delivery systems that are capable of working with families that have traditional and alternative lifestyles. The immediate family, extended family, and peer support network of one client may consist of widely diverse cultural subsystems that require separate approaches and interventions.

To meet the growing needs of persons with AIDS and their families, federal, state, and local funds, as well as grants from private foundations, are required to do the following:

■ Provide expert training for community workers.

■ Research the extent of the psychosocial, developmental, and economic problems experienced by the family and individual members.

■ Identify the unique concerns of specific cultural or minority groups.

■ Test methods of intervention.

■ Measure the educational needs of catchment areas.

■ Improve delivery systems and predict their future requirements for staff and programs.

Notes and References

1. U. Bronfenbrenner, *The Ecology of Human Development* (Cambridge, Mass.: Harvard University Press, 1979), p. 25.

2. The HTLV-III antibody test indicates if one has been exposed to the virus. The test became available in early 1985 and may be obtained commercially through the American Red Cross, local blood banks, and alternative test sites that may be located through state health departments.

3. G. H. Friedland, et al., "Lack of Transmission of HTLV-III/LAV Infection to Household Contacts of Patients with AIDS or AIDS-Related Complex with Oral Candidiasis," *New England Journal of Medicine,* 314 (February 1986), p. 344.

4. *For an example of this method, see* M. R. Goldfried and G. C. Davison, *Clinical Behavior Therapy* (New York: Holt, Rinehart & Winston, 1976), pp. 136–157.

5. *For an example of these methods, see* ibid., pp. 158–180; J. S. Wodarski, "Clinical Practice and the Social Learning Paradigm," *Social Work,* 28 (March–April 1983), pp. 154–160; A. Ellis and R. Grieger, *Handbook of Rational-Emotive Therapy* (New York: Springer Publishing Co., 1977); D. G. Langsley and D. M. Kaplan, *The Treatment of Families in Crisis* (New York: Grune & Stratton, 1968), pp. 1–66; V. E. Frankl, *The Will to Meaning* (New York: New American Library, 1969); and Frankl, *Psychotherapy and Existentialism* (New York: Simon & Schuster, 1967).

6. *For an example of this method, see* D. C. Rimm and J. Master, *Behavior Therapy* (New York: Academic Press, 1974), pp. 81–127.

7. B. E. Berstein, "Legal Needs of the Ill: The Social Worker's Role on an Interdisciplinary Team," *Health and Social Work,* 5 (August 1980), pp. 68–72.

8. D. A. Newmark, "Review of a Support Group for Patients with AIDS," *Topics in Clinical Nursing* (July 1984), pp. 38–44.

9. Ibid.

10. "Coolfont Report: A PHS Plan for Prevention and Control of AIDS and the AIDS Virus," *Public Health Reports,* 101 (July–August 1986), pp. 341–348.

6

Women and Children with AIDS

Esther Chachkes

The death of a child is an immeasurable sorrow. When the death of a child is the result of a severe illness and suffering is prolonged, we are overwhelmed and outraged that we are unable to protect our children.

Many terrible illnesses can afflict children, and social workers have witnessed the range of these tragedies. To this unfortunate list we must now add AIDS. When AIDS is the diagnosis, there is an added dimension to the devastating and shattering experience of terminal illness. Children with AIDS must contend not only with the illness itself, but with the public's fear—a reaction that promotes social isolation, rejection, and even ostracism. Vulnerability and victimization have become central themes in their lives.

Realities of the Illness

AIDS is an illness of severe morbidity and high mortality. It is transmitted in three ways: sexually, via the bloodstream (from dirty needles), and during gestation. For children, the signs and symptoms of AIDS include the failure to thrive, such recurrent bacterial infections as Otitis-media (inner ear infections); chronic intersitial pneumonitis (the only disease that the Centers for Disease Control recognize as full-blown AIDS in children and one that is not an opportunistic infection), thrush, and lymphadenopathy.[1] Because chronic inflammations and infections such as thrush and herpes make eating difficult, obtaining adequate nutrition can be a major problem. These children experience weight loss, chronic diarrhea, shortness of breath, fatigue, and impaired growth. Neurological involvement frequently leads to cognitive impairment and to regression in development or to a delay or a plateau in the achievement of developmental milestones. For example, children can regress significantly and stop feeding themselves, become incontinent if previously toilet trained, or stop walking and resort to crawling.

For their persistent bacterial infections, children with AIDS receive gamma globulin every three to four weeks, which seems to decrease the number of serious opportunistic infections and is therefore advocated as a treatment for pediatric AIDS.[2] They also may receive a range of other medications, some of which can cause allergic reactions. Intravenous feeding may be necessary to curb wasting.

Hospitalizations increase over the course of the illness. In the hospital, blood frequently is drawn, and mechanical ventilation for respiratory infections may be necessary. The experience of being in the hospital includes not only separation from one's family and home and the pain and discomfort of being sick, but all the medical routine and procedures that frighten and hurt children. In addition, children with AIDS may be subjected to enforced isolation; to nurse, physicians, and visitors who are gloved and gowned as a precaution against contracting AIDS, and to the fearful behavior of health care providers and family members. This fear, as well as the necessary precautions taken for handling blood and body fluids, can deprive these children of the intimate touching so necessary for development.

When these children are home, every cough, sneeze, episode of diarrhea, and ear infection brings the worry that they are now sicker and the infections will be more difficult to curb. Although early diagnosis and treatment can improve the quality of the children's lives somewhat and increase their life span a little, most children with AIDS die of overwhelming sepsis.

The average age of diagnosis is four to eight months, although some children have been diagnosed at birth and a few in later years. The diagnosis generally is made at six months to prevent a misdiagnosis because children may be born with genetic defects whose symptoms are similar to AIDS and that may mimic the disease.[3]

Although some children become ill after receiving blood products and blood transfusions, most children contract the virus when it is transmitted in utero or perinatally through their mothers, who may not be symptomatic or clinically ill before or during pregnancy. That AIDS is transmitted to children through their mothers is one of the most sorrowful and painful aspects of the illness. For this reason, AIDS in children cannot be discussed without discussing AIDS and families and AIDS and women. The psychosocial issues for all are inexorably bound together.

Psychosocial Problems of Women and Families

The incidence of AIDS in women is expected to rise dramatically. Women are at risk of contracting AIDS through their use of intravenous drugs or because their sexual partners are men at risk (intravenous drug abusers or bisexuals). In addition to sharing the psychosocial problems that affect all AIDS patients, women with AIDS have unique problems that are related to their social roles as mothers, specifically pregnancy and separation from their children during medical crises.

A woman who has been exposed to the virus must make critical decisions about pregnancy because although not all children who are born to at-risk women contract AIDS, many do. Should she terminate the pregnancy? Should she begin the nine-month wait to see if she and her baby will be among the lucky ones? If she fears her husband will leave her if she is ill, these decisions will be made without his support or without the support of other family members and friends who may not know about the risk factors.

For parents of children with AIDS, the mother's separation from her children is a painful consequence of long hospital stays and inadequate social supports. Parenting is further complicated for women who have AIDS; the ill mother requires sufficient social supports to help her care for herself and for her children. For the children with AIDS, separation is probably the most devastating aspect of the illness. A child's developmental age determines his or her ability to understand what is happening. Because many pediatric AIDS cases involve children under six years, separation is more critical than an awareness of their impending death.

The illness of a family member upsets all aspects of family life—social roles, economic functioning, and the relationship among family members. The family's initial struggle is to accept the diagnosis and the catastrophic nature of the illness. The family has to acknowledge long-held secrets about drug use, homosexuality, and prostitution and integrate the knowledge that lovers, a spouse, and especially children have been put at risk. Mothers of babies with AIDS, who may not be ill themselves, bear an overwhelming burden of guilt in addition to the pain and sorrow of watching their babies die.

A family has to mobilize and plan its responses to the impact of the illness on all family members, as well as to respond to the physical needs of the person with AIDS. Moreover, its members must respond quickly, even if they have not worked through their feelings to achieve understanding and acceptance. Differences in values, communication patterns, and permitted cultural responses influence the family members' reactions to the illness and how they will cope. And, most importantly, how the family behaves establishes the context in which the person with AIDS will experience the processes of his or her illness. The family's behavior is particularly significant for the child who is totally dependent on it. Some families accept the situation and find ways to meet the emotional and concrete needs of the child, but others remain too overwhelmed and overburdened to provide adequate care or to prepare for the child's death.

Although families have characteristic responses to stress, the diagnosis of AIDS generates such panic and fear that family problems and poor coping mechanisms often are magnified. Furthermore, family members are frequently conflicted about the amount of assistance they are able or willing to give. For example, family members with small children may be reluctant to help relatives with AIDS or those whose children have AIDS because they fear that AIDS will be transmitted to their children. In addition, old conflicts in the family may resurface, resulting in recriminations that obscure the best interests of the children who are involved. Although education of families about the transmission of the disease and the risk factors provides some reassurance, fear and anger often prevail.

When the person with AIDS returns to the parental home for care, feelings of dependence and loss of control and autonomy, usually part of a severe illness, are aggravated. In families, in which matriarchal patterns are dominant, the return to the protection of the mother can be conflictual as well as nurturing. The Hispanic or black grandmother, for example, may feel obligated to assume a more significant caregiving role with the children than does the mother.

Despite the overwhelming burdens that families must shoulder to care for a patient with AIDS, most do not abandon their loved ones. Affection and concern prevail more often than does rejection.

Abuse of Intravenous Drugs

The majority of mothers of babies with AIDS are intravenous drug abusers or the sexual partners of such abusers. The large number of abusers, particularly in urban areas, presents an alarming number of potential AIDS sufferers. This population is young, and many have two or more children.

Because intravenous drug abusers with AIDS are predominantly from minority groups, poverty and discrimination are often central to their lives. As a result, their social resources may be limited, unrealiable, and inconsistent and their use of health care services sporadic and crisis oriented. Furthermore, their behavior tends to be self-destructive, and their poor self-management skills obstruct their compliance with medical treatment.

These characteristics of intravenous drug users create tension between health care providers and patients and make it difficult for them to trust each other or to develop feelings of goodwill. Families with an AIDS patient must have a complex relationship with the health care system because they are dependent on it. They must come to feel that they are in caring hands and must perceive health care providers as humane and sensitive. If previous experiences raise the expectation of a hostile reception, it takes sensitivity, patience, and skill to help them accept and comply with medical routines and treatment.[4]

Case Illustrations

Perhaps the best way to discuss the range of psychosocial issues in working with AIDS patients is through case examples. The following two cases involve children—as persons with AIDS and as children of parents with AIDS. These cases, which were taken from the caseloads of social workers at Montefiore Medical Center and the Albert Einstein College of Medicine, New York City, illustrate the complex needs generated by the illness as well as the multifaceted work that characterizes social work interventions. The cases are real, although some of the details have been changed to protect confidentiality.[5]

Marion

Marion came to the clinic when she was first experiencing symptoms that raised the possibility of AIDS. She was a 27-year-old Hispanic woman who lived with her two children (aged 3 and 4) and her three brothers in an apartment in the Bronx, New York. Both her parents were dead; she had moved in with her brothers after she left her husband several months before her first appointment at the clinic. Her husband who was an intravenous drug abuser and may have been bisexual, died shortly after she left him, probably from AIDS, although this diagnosis was never confirmed.

Marion was not a drug addict and had never used drugs. She had contracted AIDS because she was the sexual partner of an infected male. Of her three brothers, two were addicts, who gave her and her children no emotional or concrete support. Her third brother, who was gay, died soon after she moved in, also of AIDS.

Marion had two sisters. Both were married and one was pregnant. They were afraid of catching the disease from her and would not see her. In addition, their husbands strongly objected to any contact with her.

Marion had left school at an early age. She was illiterate, never worked, and was supported by public assistance all her life. Marion's social situation deteriorated rapidly after the death of her brother. She lived in fear of eviction and violence from her two drug-addicted brothers. She had few supports and was depressed and isolated. The risk of suicide was real.

Marion was desperately in need of emotional support and called the social worker as often as three times a day. She also needed help in managing her day-to-day affairs. She had few budgeting skills and was disorganized and overwhelmed by the smallest task. The social worker arranged for a home attendant, who stabilized her situation somewhat. Marion was encouraged to attend a patient-family group that met weekly; she often brought her children to these meetings.

Marion's main concern, which preoccupied her during the course of her illness, was the future of her children. Before AIDS had weakened her, she did her best to be a parent to them and to provide for their needs. At one point, she attempted to enroll them in a Head Start program because she wanted to give them a better life than she had. The program, knowing of their father's death from AIDS, refused to admit the children, although the children showed no signs of AIDS.

Marion raced against time to make the arrangements she thought would carry out her hopes that her children's lives would be protected after she died. The social worker helped her reach out to distant cousins who were willing to accept the children. These cousins were a young, stable family with children of their own. Marion was helped to prepare a will that was witnessed by the social worker and signed in the presence of a hospital administrator who was also a notary public.

Soon afterward, Marion became increasingly weak and remained bedridden until she died. The children were cared for by the home attendant with some help from Marion's cousins. After Marion's death, the home attendant brought the children to live with their paternal grandmother, who requested custody. The grandmother, in keeping with the Hispanic culture, considered it her right and obligation to raise her son's children. A court battle ensued. The social workers were drawn into the interfamilial issues even after Marion's death. Numerous family meetings were held, which included religious leaders and lawyers. A temporary compromise was reached in which the cousins would have custody of the children and the grandmother would have visiting rights. Although the case is still in court, it is likely that this arrangement will prevail because it was Marion's wish and because the grandmother is old, poor, and unable to handle the children.

Carol

Carol was a 3-year-old Hispanic child, who lived with her mother, a single parent, and three siblings (a four-year-old sister, a nine-year-old brother who was retarded, and a 10-year-old sister). She was diagnosed as having ARC following numerous ear infections and pneumonia that was difficult to control. Within three months, full-blown AIDS was diagnosed. Carol spent 4½ months in the hospital before she died.

Carol's mother, Mrs. S, was a healthy, asymptomatic carrier of the HIV virus, who probably had been infected by Carol's father—an intravenous drug abuser who lived with the family only sporadically. Mrs. S was isolated and had few friends or community supports. She was afraid to leave her children with friends or neighbors because of the erratic behavior of her retarded son, who was a danger to himself and others. Mrs. S needed considerable help to deal with Carol's illness and to learn how to care for her sick child.

The social worker managed to obtain services from the Office of the Handicapped so that the retarded son could enroll in a special education program; the 4-year-old daughter was enrolled in a preschool class. These arrangements allowed Mrs. S to visit Carol more frequently and relieved the burden somewhat. However, home health aides who were brought in refused to stay because of the AIDS environment and the chaotic family situation.

Carol developed brain cancer but was unable to return home even for the brief time that her medical condition permitted because the apartment was rat infested and her father's increased use of drugs made him abusive to the children. After discussions with the Department of Health, the decision was made to keep Carol in the hospital. Mrs. S began to visit her less frequently because she was desperately attempting to deal with the deteriorating situation at home. Carol's despair over their seperation was heartbreaking, and she was inconsolable. At times, unable to cope, Mrs. S left her other children alone. She was reported for child neglect, which added to her misery. The father was finally encouraged to leave to join his family in Puerto Rico, which made it possible for Mrs. S to visit the hospital more frequently during the last three months of Carol's life. Carol died in her mother's arms. Her funeral was arranged by the social worker because Mrs. S was destitute, depressed, and exhausted. After the funeral, Mrs. S did not respond to the social worker's calls and letters offering further help.

Although these cases are typical of those found in the caseloads of social workers who treat AIDS patients, the situations are not new. Social workers have always worked with mothers who have passed on genetic defects to their children, who have parented while terminally ill, and who have suffered multiple deaths in a family, and they often have seen how a magnitude of social, economic, and emotional sorrows can converge on one unfortunate family. What is unique to families with AIDS, however, is that this suffering is experienced in a context of public condemnation and fear that frequently results in the withdrawal by others of emphathic support, which is needed to buffer the impact of the illness and to strengthen coping responses.

Both cases illustrate most of the important psychosocial factors associated with AIDS:

■ AIDS is a terminal illness with a debilitating course that affects young people.

■ Fear, hopelessness, and the entire range of emotions associated with a terminal illness are made more dramatic because they exist in the context of stigma.

■ The disapproval of family and friends often leads to isolation.

■ Persons with AIDS experience multiple losses—of social role, emotional support, physical strength, self-sufficiency, a sexual life, and of others who also may have died of the illness.

■ AIDS patients suffer guilt for having exposed lovers, children, and spouses to the disease through past behaviors and sexual preferences.

■ Most women and children with AIDS are poor and victims of discrimination.

■ AIDS causes deep suffering in a family and disrupts its equilibrium.

■ For many intravenous drug abusers, chaotic family situations provide only inconsistent or unreliable social supports.

■ For health care givers and the health care system, AIDS is labor intensive, expensive, and emotionally draining.

■ The rigidity of bureautic organizations impedes the patients' access to services.

■ Personnel in many of the social institutions and public agencies that deal with persons with AIDS react to these victims with stigma and fear, further alienating them when they need these connections the most.

Social Work Intervention

Social work interventions are the most helpful when they reflect the profession's emphasis on person-in-situation. Services are more effective when they assist the person with AIDS to maintain an ongoing and positive interaction with the health care and social service systems. Services that support the coping of family members and the cohesiveness of the family avoid the risk of the impersonal care that is prevalent in discharge planning. Family-centered social services are thus the critical focus of helping.

To assist AIDS patients and their families with the range of social and health services they need to cope with AIDS and to protect their quality of life, social workers must be involved in a variety of professional activities. These activities include advocacy, interagency linkages and liaisons, the development of community services, case management, discharge planning, and crisis intervention.

The following sections describe the needs of AIDS patients and their families and the many problems they face in obtaining services. Social workers can assist with some problems and can humanize the bureaucratic processes that must be negotiated to obtain resources, but they cannot help in all instances. Some resources are simply too scarce and thus remain unavailable to many patients who desperately need them.

Housing

Public fear about the transmission of AIDS and other public health concerns have made it especially difficult for persons with AIDS to obtain housing in an already-tight housing market. Those who have lost their housing because they cannot work or have been abandoned by lovers and family members have few places to go. High rents make housing, particularly larger units appropriate for families, unaffordable. In New York City, persons with AIDS cannot be housed in public shelters because of the living conditions and shared bathrooms. Welfare hotels and group homes will not accept patients who are visibly ill. Landlords have been known to evict persons with AIDS and certainly are reluctant to rent to them. Although New York City has organized some scatter-bed housing, this effort barely begins to address the number of units required. The New York City Human Resources Administration has been able to preserve some housing by assisting with rent payments and, at times, extending the public assistance allowance for shelter. However, even this housing may cease to be available to families once the person with AIDS has died and the enriched allocation is terminated.

As a result of the housing problem, many persons with AIDS have lingered in hospitals, spending the precious time when they are less sick in an institution rather than in the community with family and friends. This is a particularly tragic situation when children are involved.

The only housing that is available to many mothers and children is overcrowded and inadequate, which places untold burdens on families and friends who are attempting to care for them. In addition, this housing often cannot accommodate live-in home health aides because there simply is no room or the conditions are too chaotic.

Income Maintenance

In many families, working women provide the economic foundation for the family. When they contract AIDS or are called on to provide primary care to children or adults with AIDS, they may not be able to continue to work. The impact on the family's economic well-being of these women's unemployment is severe. Therefore, social workers must help these women to obtain public assistance, through early intervention and advocacy, so their families can survive economically. They must do so because the complexities and insensitivities of overburdened public agencies are difficult enough to negotiate when one is well but virtually impossible when one is ill.

When the person with AIDS is eligible for disability benefits from social security because of a work history, there are other problems. Although these benefits generally are higher than public assistance benefits, medical benefits under Medicare are not available until two consecutive years after social security disability checks have been received. Obviously, AIDS patients require immediate medical benefits because many do not even survive for two years. If there is no other health insurance, the person with AIDS must apply for Medicaid and public assistance, whose benefits are lower. Furthermore, ARC patients are not eligible for disability benefits under social security because they are not considered to be as disabled as AIDS patients.

Long Term and Hospice Care

Families with AIDS need a respite from caregiving, which can be provided, when appropriate, through in-home or in-hospital hospice care. Although many patients welcome hospice services, young persons in particular find it difficult to tolerate the hospice philosophy, which promotes acceptance of the inevitability of death from AIDS. In addition, hospice treatment is primarily palliative, and many young persons want active treatment until the end. If the requirement to accept the terminal nature of the illness were less rigidly enforced by the hospices, young people would benefit from these services.

When intensive nursing and medical care are needed but inappropriate in an acute care setting, long-term care in skilled nursing facilities should be provided. However, most skilled nursing facilities are reluctant to admit persons with AIDS, and only a few long-term nursing homes have been made available to AIDS patients.

Home Care

Almost all persons with AIDS require home care services at some point in their illness, particularly between hospitalizations when they are feeling better. Toward the end of their illness, many cannot be supported in the community without full-day or round-the-clock services. The cost of these services is substantial. Aides must be specially trained and the hours of service increased quickly to protect the patient's ability to remain at home or to leave the hospital.

In New York City, as elsewhere, health care and social service systems in the community are separate and have different requirements for eligibility. In addition, the division of responsibility among a variety of human service agencies and the lack of interagency coordination has made it a nightmare for social workers to plan for community support services and discharge from a hospital.

New York City has attempted to improve this situation by establishing an AIDS Crisis Intervention Service to coordinate services among its various agencies. In March 1986, the AIDS Case Management Unit of the New York City Human Resources Administration became the sole intake point for all Medicaid-funded home care services for persons with AIDS. In addition, the unit assists persons with AIDS to become eligible for other entitlement programs and to resolve housing problems. These actions have lessened, to some extent, the victimization of persons with AIDS by inflexible, confusing, and unresponsive systems.

Child Care and Foster Care

Mothers of children with AIDS need babysitters for their other children so that the mothers can visit their afflicted children in the hospital or take them for the many medical treatments they require. If the mothers are ill themselves, they need other people to take over the care of their children. This additional child care help is essential if the family is to stay together.

For children with AIDS whose families cannot or will not care for them, foster care is essential. Without foster care, these children remain in the hospital until they die. However, foster homes are difficult to find because of the fear of many people that these children will transmit AIDS and the reluctance to care for a dying child. Those foster parents that can be found need special services to maintain these homes, as well as enriched allocations to cover the increased costs of supplies, transportation, and other essentials.

Counseling and Mental Health

Counseling and mental health services are critical, especially for families in the childbearing years when sex and pregnancy are fraught with danger and fear. Adolescents, in particular, need guidance because AIDS in the family can intensify their normal feelings of resentment and rebelliousness. And, of course, sexual counseling and education about drug abuse are essential.

Children in families with AIDS may lose parents, siblings, and other close family members. Young children have difficulty relating their feelings to events. However, they react to the sadness, anxiety, and fear of family members and the adults' preoccupation with the ill member and their feelings of being emotionally overwhelmed. This situation, along with repeated separations from parents, can leave the children feeling frightened and unprotected. Lacking verbal and cognitive skills, they may act out their fears and sadness with unacceptable behavior, which places yet another strain on the adults. Furthermore, if the children do not appear to react, the adults may minimize the children's problems because they assume that the children are too young to understand. Depending on their age and developmental level, children can regress and lose recently attained developmental skills, such as toilet training. They may show disturbances in sleeping, eating, and socializing and become clinging and demanding or withdrawn. Family counseling can help the adults understand these reactions and help all the family members deal with them.

Legal Interventions and Child Custody

Legal assistance has been critical in two important areas: prospective planning for health care decisions and child custody arrangements. Prospective planning for health care decisions has been made more imperative with the increasing evidence of neurological complications associated with AIDS. When a person is no longer able to participate in decisions regarding care, documented preferences for treatment via the durable power of an attorney or a living will can lift the burden placed on health care providers and families.

Many young mothers are consumed with anxiety about the child custody arrangements for their children after their death. The issue is complex. The mothers may have had several children with different fathers or the fathers' drug addiction, violent behavior, or lack of involvement may make them unacceptable custodians even though they may have a legal claim on the children. In addition, the fathers may also be ill with AIDS.

A mother may decide on custodians who are peripheral to the family because she perceives distant relatives or friends as being more stable than her immediate relatives. This decision can offend close relatives, particularly the grandmother, who may assume that she should be the responsible custodian. Conflict over future custody can result in a resurrection of old family conflicts in which children, as always, are caught in the middle. To avoid such a situation, social workers, clergy, lawyers, and others should sensitively intervene in the family system early enough to complete the arrangements before the mother is too ill to participate.

Delivery of Medical Care and Health Education

In medical settings, the routine and accepted rotations of staff, particularly physicians, are especially difficult for persons with AIDS. Those patients who do not have an attending physician in the hospital may have to relate to many different physicians, as may those whose hospitalization is prolonged for acute care episodes. Rotations of physicians in clinics create a similar situation. This pattern of multiple physicians detracts from the ongoing support and continuity of care that are needed to manage an illness such as AIDS.

Medical care is problem oriented and focused mainly on curative efforts. The AIDS crisis, however, has prompted an increasing number of preventive efforts, largely through health education and information programs. These programs, which are offered in health care facilities as well as in the community, are targeted to the promotion of safe sex and the decreased use of drugs.

Health education is more effective when open, explicit discussions of homosexuality and bisexuality, sexual practices, promiscuous sex, and birth control and abortion take place. Social workers play a critical role in promoting these discussions with individuals or groups and in counseling women who face these complex issues.

Most seropositive women come from minority groups in which macho cultures prevail. In these cultures, bisexual activity is often denied. Therefore, it is imperative that these women receive the help and support that make it possible for them to confront their husbands and lovers about previous sexual practices, the use of condoms, and sexual activities that should be avoided.

In addition, seropositive women must decide if pregnancy should be prevented or terminated. To make this difficult decision, women may need to discuss their fears and decisions, their concerns about religious and cultural consequences, and the reactions of family members, husbands, lovers, and others. Social work counseling can offer a significant service by providing support to these overburdened women, as well as to those who are trying to get off or stay off drugs.

Although most efforts are now targeted to at-risk women, it would be a tragic mistake to limit public health education to this designated group. All women need to know the facts about the issues involved in AIDS and should be encouraged to take a strong stand about the sexual behavior that will promote their well-being and protect their health.

Social Policy

With the expected increases in the number of AIDS/ARC patients and people infected with HIV virus, AIDS represents one of the nation's most significant public health problems. All health professionals, particularly social workers whose professional involvement centers on the care of vulnerable populations, will work with persons with AIDS some time in their professional lives.

The demand for intensive medical interventions and health care and the costs of these interventions will continue to rise, as will the need for social support services. Obtaining the variety of needed and appropriate services is a difficult task. Social programs, as they are currently constructed, often impede the development of a flexible and logically managed system of care. Fragmented systems with gaps and discontinuities in services predominate. Added to this situation are the negative social attitudes and stereotypes toward minorities, the poor, gays, and drug addicts. Furthermore, the ideological distinctions between those who are deserving and those who are not have surfaced in the public's responses to AIDS.

Despite the overwhelming social needs of so many persons with AIDS and their families, the resulting demands on public resources, and the anticipated escalation in the incidence of AIDS, it appears unlikely that current social policy will lead to long-term planning or to a coordinated and comprehensive response. On the contrary, national health and social policy has been influenced by an emphasis on cost containment, deregulation, and the limited role of the federal government in public health and social programs. Responsibility has shifted to local governments and to the private sector, both of which clearly are unable to carry the extensive burden of care that AIDS patients require. The AIDS crisis emphasizes the reality that national problems must be addressed on a national level. Although the influence of current political and economic factors on the allocation of funds for the development of public health programs may seriously compromise the ability of social workers and health care providers to maintain adequate medical and community support services, the experience with AIDS presents the opportunity to reexamine attitudes and priorities. It is hoped that the commitment to a more socially intelligent and caring response will be strengthened and will lead to a reconsideration of current social policies.

Notes and References

1. *For a more complete discussion of the medical aspects of pediatric AIDS, see* M. F. Rogers, "AIDS in Children, A Review of the Clinical Epidemiologic and Public Health Aspects," *Pediatric Infectious Disease,* 4 (May 1985), pp. 230–236; M. Bolard and T. D. B. Gaskill, "Managing AIDS in Children"

MCN 9 (November–December 1984), pp. 384–389; and K. M. Shannon and A. G. Animann, "Acquired Immune Deficiency Syndrome in Childhood," *Journal of Pediatrics,* 106 (February 1985), pp. 332–342.

2. Shannon and Animann, "Acquired Immune Deficiency Syndrome in Childhood," p. 339; and A. Rubenstein, Editorial, *American Journal of Diseases of Children,* 137 (September 1983), p. 827.

3. Some congenital immunodeficiency disorders include DiGeorge syndrome, Lieskatt-Aldrich syndrome, ataxia-telangiectasia, and severe combined immunodeficiency. *See* M. F. Rogers, "AIDS in Children: A Review of the Clinical Epidemiologic and Public Health Aspects," *Pediatric Infectious Disease,* 4 (May 1985), p. 233.

4. *For a discussion of AIDS and addiction, see* E. Drucker, "AIDS and Addictions in New York City," *American Journal of Drug and Alcohol Abuse,* 12, Nos. 1 and 2 (1986), pp. 165–181.

5. Both cases involve Hispanic families; they were chosen because over 90 percent of the AIDS patients who are treated at the two institutions from which the cases were taken are black or Hispanic. The author is indebted to Lauren Gordon and Anita Septimus for sharing these case illustrations with her.

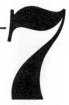

Identifying and Meeting the Needs of Minority Clients with AIDS

Sally Jue

One of this country's most distinguishing features is its diverse and ever-growing ethnic population. The three largest ethnic minority groups are blacks, Asians, and Hispanics. According to the 1980 census, these three ethnic groups make up over 28 percent of the U.S. population.[1] However, people from these groups make up 40 percent of all adults with AIDS and 81 percent of all children with AIDS.[2]

Whether born in this country or elsewhere, ethnic minority people retain in varying degrees, aspects of their culture and language. Furthermore, there are differences within each group. Black Americans who are raised in the urban North differ from those who are raised in the rural South and those who have immigrated from the West Indies and Africa. Hispanics come from many countries in Central and South American and the Caribbean, in addition to those who were born here. And Asians, both those who were born in this country and those who emigrated, represent over 100 languages and dialects from nearly 40 countries and territories. The needs of these groups are as diverse as are their ways of expressing themselves and coping with problems. Therefore, interventions that are appropriate for white Americans often are ineffective with clients from these minority groups.

In working with ethnic minority clients with AIDS and their families, it is essential to have some understanding of the clients' cultural values and how they influence behavior. Unfortunately, the issues that surface are ones that have been well hidden and rarely researched. Thus, there is virtually no information on the attitudes of minority groups toward gay and bisexual behaviors in their communities. Furthermore, there is little information on the prevention and treatment of substance abuse with minority clients or the effect of the stresses of acculturation and coping with numerous societally imposed stigmas on family relationships and the development of identity and self-esteem.

The material presented in this article is based on articles on minority families in the literature. It also is based on extensive interviews that the author conducted with minority clients with AIDS and their families; minority gay volunteers; minority health and social service professionals who have worked with AIDS patients in minority communities, the gay community, AIDS programs, and drug treatment programs; and on the responses of minority people to AIDS education seminars presented by the author.[3] Empirical data to support many of the positions expressed in this article are unavailable because this is a new field of inquiry on which data are still being gathered.

Information about AIDS is not widespread in minority communities, and what has been circulated has often met with denial or apathy. Much of the information has been culturally inappropriate. Written materials are of no use to those who cannot read English or who cannot read at all. Much of the information is too technical or sexually explicit according to the standard of minority cultures. The stigma attached to AIDS is so great that communities that already feel stigmatized are unwilling to take on another one by admitting they need to be concerned about AIDS.

Attitudes Toward AIDS

Asians tend to view AIDS as a Western disease brought on by the high-risk behaviors of Americans and other Western people. Furthermore, the small number of Asians, here and in Asian countries, who have been diagnosed as having AIDS reinforces this belief. The Asians believe that if one adheres to Asian cultural norms, there is no need to be concerned about AIDS.

Hispanics also tend to view AIDS as an American problem. Many have heard of AIDS but have little information, other than, as one client put it, "it's a sleazy disease." Sexual behavior is not a socially acceptable topic of conversation among most Asians and Hispanics, so discussing how AIDS is transmitted may be uncomfortable for them.

The black community continues to struggle with its feelings about AIDS. Although blacks make up 25 percent of all AIDS cases, they are still angry, resentful, suspicious, and sometimes defensive about AIDS.[4] Because AIDS is believed to have originated in Africa and, until last year, Haitians were considered a separate high-risk group, many blacks feel that another stigma has been foisted on them in the underlying message that there may be something intrinsic to blacks that makes them responsible for the origin and spread of the disease.

Homosexuality

Admitting that AIDS affects minority communities also means acknowledging the existence of homosexuality, bisexuality, and the use of intravenous drugs. When a person is diagnosed with AIDS, it is difficult to continue to hide his or her lifestyle or behavior. The stress of maintaining secrets, the anguish of deciding whether to inform one's family, and the possible consequences of such a disclosure are dilemmas that all persons with AIDS must face. In working with minority clients, it is necessary to examine these issues within the cultural context of each group.

As of June 30, 1986, the Centers for Disease Control reported that 107 Asians, 3,101 Hispanics, and 5,404 blacks had been diagnosed with AIDS. The proportion of men in these groups of AIDS victims who acknowledged that they were gay or bisexual was: Asians, 78 percent; Hispanics, 55 percent; and blacks, 46 percent.[5] These percentages probably are deflated because other men with AIDS in these groups may have chosen not to reveal that they were gay or bisexual for fear of rejection by families and communities or because they were unable to accept these behaviors in themselves. Therefore, more accurate information can be obtained by asking clients about specific behaviors, rather than whether they have labeled themselves as gay or bisexual.

There is little information on gay and bisexual men in these minority groups. Many are hidden in their communities, where taboos against homosexuality appear stronger than in white communities. Ethnic concerns take precedence over sexual orientation because one is socialized into a culture from birth, and sexual identity develops later. Ethnicity is a fundamental part of a minority client's identity, and those who have emotional, familial, or economic ties to their ethnic community are more likely to conform to group norms. It is a struggle to integrate minority and American cultures but, if one is gay, the process is more difficult and complex.

In all minority communities, homosexuality is taboo. Most consider homosexuals to be men trying to be women or as engaging in isolated sexual behaviors that they can choose to do or not to do. Homosexuality often is viewed as perverted and obscene, a disease to be cured, or a sin against God and nature. Nearly all minority clients voiced feelings of isolation and lamented the absence of positive role models, in their communities. The absence of a supportive environment and the low visibility of minority gay people has helped perpetuate the perception that homosexuality is a white American phenomenon. There is no evidence of gay pride in minority communities. Thus, to be gay often requires one to choose to join the white gay community or to remain isolated in one's own community. What are some of the cultural factors that contribute to this situation?

Attitudes of Asians

In Asian cultures, the family (and often the extended family) is the most important social unit and remains the primary socializing agent throughout one's life. One's behavior is a reflection on the entire family—not just the individual. Therefore, one shows one's love and loyalty to the family by fulfilling the required role expectations. In return, the family provides support and security.

When sons marry, they are not starting new families but continuing the existing one.[6] Because the needs of the family take precedence over those of the individual, great pressure is put on sons to marry and have children. Unmarried children are expected to live with their parents and to care for them. Although the oldest son is favored, he also has more responsibilities and family obligations.[7] He is expected to be a role model for his younger siblings and to be the caretaker of the family if the father is unable to fulfill that role.

Conformity to group norms is valued, and anything different is suspect. In many Asian languages, the word for "homosexual" also means "deviant." Many Asians believe that homosexuality is the result of "bad blood"—an affliction to be cured—or a Western corruption. In such Asian countries as the Philippines, more visible homosexuals tend to be overly effeminate or transvestites. They are tolerated as eccentric, amusing, and harmless.

In Asian cultures, it is inconceivable that a man who is not overtly feminine could be gay. However, in most Asian countries, being openly gay in the community means public humiliation not only for the individual, but for his family as well because it implies that his parents have failed to raise him properly and that he is rejecting his family and culture. If the child is an only son, being gay also means the end of the family. Thus, rejection of gay men by the community and the need to protect family relations force many gay Asians out of the community or further into the closet.

Attitudes of Hispanics

The family is also central in Hispanic cultures, and the extended family often includes godparents.[8] There is a high level of interaction among family members, and the family is viewed as a source of support, security, and strength. Family functions are important, as are children because they validate and cement the marriage; occasionally the bond between the mother and her children is stronger than the marital bond.[9] As with Asians, an individual's behavior is a reflection of the entire family, and unmarried children are expected to live with their parents to help care for them.

Hispanics are heavily influenced by Roman Catholicism. Although many are not religious, they are still cultural Roman Catholics. Thus, the Roman Catholic Church's views on homosexuality, divorce, abortion, birth control, families and children, guilt as a means of social control, and sacrificing in this life with the hope of a better afterlife are important considerations in planning educational programs about AIDS and in delivering services.

Homosexuality is viewed as a sin against God, counterproductive to having offspring, or just "not being right in the head." In Puerto Rico, gay men are often referred to as *locas*—the feminine form of the noun crazy person. In South America, gay bars exist only in large metropolitan areas and are discreet. Some clients reported that, in general conversations, their parents told them they would kill or disown a gay son. Ironically, in most Hispanic countries, certain gay-associated sexual behaviors are acceptable and even considered macho. Anal and oral sex between two men is acceptable only for the anal active, oral receptive partner. That person is just "getting off" or indulging in another form of masturbation. For him, there is nothing emotional or erotic about the experience. The anal receptive, oral active person is the *loca*.

Nearly all the foreign-born openly gay Hispanics interviewed by the author stated that they were "closeted" in their own countries and did not come out until they came to the United States. Some were married in these countries or had had sexual relationships with women in the hopes of proving to themselves that they were not really gay. Greater educational or economic opportunities were a pretext for coming to the United States, where they believed they could live a more open gay lifestyle without having to reveal themselves to their families.

Attitudes of Blacks

The scars of slavery and the years of blatant racism and discrimination since the abolition of slavery continue to leave their imprint on the black community. Because the African culture was destroyed and black family relationships were not acknowledged, black Americans developed a strong sense of group survival that they passed on to subsequent generations.

Many black families have strong kinship bonds that may include extended family members and close friends. Because of their history of oppression, blacks "often expose children to the harsher aspects of reality earlier to prepare them to cope."[10] This exposure can lead to emotional precocity and possibly earlier sexual exploration and development.[11] The black culture allows more flexible sex roles than do the Asian or Hispanic cultures, so there is more room for a wider range of sexual expression. Sex roles and sexual behavior are more rigid and well defined in the Asian and Hispanic cultures.

Protestant churches play an important role in black communities. They are a source of support and a means of achieving status and leadership in the community.[12] Black churches, like most others, disapprove of homosexuality.

The fear of racial genocide lingers on, so having children is important. An added complication is the large number of incarcerated black men and the higher mortality rate of those who are not. Role expectations for black men, then, can become highly politicized. Being gay is another threat to the survival of the group.

"Coming Out"

"Coming out," or revealing oneself, as a gay person is a traumatic experience for many, but, to minority clients, it may mean having to leave their communities and forgoing a part of their ethnic identity. However, many gay minority clients have found that they were not accepted by the gay white community either. Those who are discreet in their own communities and do not openly confront the issue are better tolerated because people can then believe what they choose. Others do not come out until they have formed a strong alternate support system, and many others remain in the closet.

Gay minority clients with AIDS who inform their families of their homosexuality before they are diagnosed do not have to go through the additional trauma of revealing themselves when they are diagnosed. Some families have been rejecting, and others have been supportive but will not reveal their son's lifestyle or diagnosis to others in the community. Families generally have little understanding of what it means to be gay and may blame themselves for their son having AIDS because they failed to raise him to be hetereosexual. Some families try to find other reasons why their sons contracted AIDS; to keep peace in the family, their sons will "admit" to more "socially acceptable" ways of acquiring AIDS, such as the use of intravenous drugs or the frequenting of prostitutes. Many clients never tell their families of their behaviors or diagnosis; they say they have cancer or pneumonia.

Bisexuality and the Feelings of Wives

The need to maintain cultural values and group survival exert strong pressures on minority men to marry and have children. For those men who are more dependent on or emotionally tied to their ethnic community, bisexuality is an alternative to being gay. A significant but undocumented number of minority clients did not find marriage and casual affairs with men mutually exclusive activities. The prevailing belief is that is they fulfill their family and community obligations and are discreet, they are free to have affairs with other men. If the wives know, they are often silent and tolerate the affairs, preferring to invest more of their energies into their children. The wives describe their husbands as good providers, fathers, and sexual partners, who care about their families.

Because of the fear of exposing their double lives, these men tend to have multiple anonymous sexual contacts outside their communities. They are the most likely to deny the gay or bisexual label or to admit they have sex with men. Most wives have no idea of their husbands' extramarital affairs until their spouses are diagnosed with AIDS. Then, the effects are devastating.

The wives of bisexual men with AIDS experience anger, betrayal, loss of trust, and fear for their health and that of their young children who may have been conceived while the father was infectious. They also feel inadequate and ashamed—that they are failures as wives. Normally, these women would turn to their families and friends for support but, because of the stigma and their sense of shame, they cannot bring themselves to discuss their feelings with anyone in the community. They would suffer social ostracism if they abandoned an ill husband and, if they are monolingual, would have difficulty finding support elsewhere. It is equally difficult for these women to decide how much to reveal to their adult children. Thus, most of them shoulder the burden of keeping the truth to themselves in addition to caring for their spouses and families with little or no support. To compound the tragedy, some of these women will eventually be diagnosed with AIDS.

In minority communities, 3 percent of each of the black, Hispanic, and Asian cases of AIDS have been transmitted by heterosexual contact.[13] Most of these cases have been women, married or single. In the Asian and Hispanic cultures, women are not supposed to have sexual relations unless they are married; those who do, if found out, are considered a disgrace to their families. It is also less acceptable for women to use intravenous drugs. Therefore, minority women with AIDS are reluctant to tell their families because they are afraid of being disowned for the behaviors that led them to contract AIDS as well as for having the disease.

An additional problem for minority women is the lack of information not only about AIDS but about birth control and other sexually transmitted diseases. Those women who have access to birth control devices do not always use them; to be prepared means that one has considered having sexual relations, which is something that only "bad" girls do. Furthermore, many minority women do not believe in abortion for cultural or religious reasons. Thus, if they get pregnant, minority women with AIDS are likely to give birth to children who will eventually develop AIDS. To date, 60 percent of all children with AIDS have been black and 21 percent have been Hispanic; most of them acquired AIDS in utero from their infected mothers.[14]

Drug Abuse

About 85 percent of all the people who contracted AIDS from using intravenous drugs have been from minority groups, primarily black and Hispanic.[15] Drugs provide immediate gratification and distraction from the hopelessness of many users' lives. They also create a sense of belonging in young people, especially those who are more acculturated than their parents and are experiencing cultural clashes at home. If one or both parents uses drugs or alcohol to cope, the risk of their children following suit increases. Drug abusers who are poor are more likely than are affluent abusers to share needles or frequent shooting galleries, since needles are difficult to obtain.

For some parents, the abuse of drugs and alcohol is a part of life. Other parents lack knowledge about drugs and drug use, do not often discuss the use of these substances, and are insecure about handling such situations because they did not have to deal with them in their former country or their own upbringing.

Alcohol and nonintravenous drugs contribute indirectly to the spread of AIDS. When one is under the influence of such substances, one's judgment is impaired and the likelihood of engaging in unsafe sex increases. Drug also are used to heighten sensations or, for those who are ambivalent, a way to overcome inhibitions and later to disclaim responsibility for the behavior ("It wasn't my fault because I was high"). One client stated that he had sex with men only when he was high because he could not handle it any other way. Because of the added stress involved in being gay or bisexual and the prevalence of drugs in some minority communities, minority people are at a greater risk of contracting AIDS from a combination of drug use and sexual behavior.

Obstacles to the Use of Mental Health Services

When persons from ethnic minority groups have problems, they rarely share them with strangers. Instead, they seek assistance from family members, friends, family physicians, ministers, priests, or folk healers or herbalists. They think that mental health services are only for "crazy people." The stigma of AIDS and its associated high-risk behaviors make them reluctant to seek help within their communities yet unsure of what support and understanding, if any, is available outside their communities, especially if they speak little or no English.

Often minority clients do not know what social workers do or what counseling is and do not think it makes sense to pay someone to listen to them talk about their problems. They are more familiar with the medical model in which physicians prescribe medication for symptoms. Asians and Hispanics, who have a greater tendency to somatize problems than do blacks, find it especially difficult to differentiate between somatic complaints and the symptoms of AIDS-related infections.[16] Headaches; nausea; poor appetite; and changes in sleep patterns, libido, and concentration may be organic or emotional, so it is important to work closely with the client's physician.

It is more useful for the social worker to explain how he or she can assist a client than to describe what therapy is. Minority clients prefer a more concrete, directive, problem-solving approach with immediate results.[17] Information and referral, advocacy, and benefits and concrete services are their initial needs, rather than discussions of their feelings and life histories.

Following through on concrete tasks will reinforce the clients' perception that the social worker understands their needs and can be helpful. Afterwards, they will be more receptive to sharing personal feelings. Because clients with AIDS believe they cannot go to their families for help, they are forced to seek assistance elsewhere. It is the first time that many of them have have to negotiate systems outside their communities. If they speak little or no English, the task is overwhelming.

Trust

Trust is essential to building a successful relationship with minority clients who often are unsure of how well workers from different ethnic backgrounds will understand them or who find it difficult to express themselves in English. Minority clients perceive the white gay community as having the most knowledge about and resources to cope with AIDS but are unsure if that community will accept and support them.

To build trust, all the minority AIDS clients who were interviewed stated their need to feel that the worker cared about them as individuals and that the relationship was personal—not strictly business. What white workers may view as unprofessional self-disclosures or useless chitchat is important to minority clients.

The first sessions may be spent on concrete tasks and sharing information about each other, rather than taking a detailed personal history. Sharing information equalizes the power differential in the relationship and makes the relationship more personal. Minority clients often ask social workers, directly or indirectly, if they are gay, married or have children, where they grew up, or why they chose to work with people with AIDS. Information about a worker enables the client to decide whether he or she can trust the worker to understand his or her different needs. With clients who are undocumented residents, trust is even more important because of their fear of deportation to countries in which medical care for AIDS patients is often inadequate or unavailable and the social climate is less accepting.

Confidentiality

Another important concern of minority clients is confidentiality. Some minority clients may be living with parents or have parents visiting who may know the diagnosis but not the high-risk behavior involved. During home visits or work with the family, it is important for the social worker to clarify with the client what he or she wishes others to know. Perhaps some members of the family know and others do not. Most families are loathe to tell their friends or even other family members about their child's diagnosis of AIDS for fear of social ostracism. Minority clients also may want to know about confidentiality and record-keeping policies because of their additional fear that high-risk behaviors and a diagnosis of AIDS may jeopardize their immigration status.

Social workers also must be prepared to tackle their racist, homophobic, and discriminatory attitudes as well as their clients' experiences with racism, homophobia, and discrimination. An understanding of how these issues affect minority clients' self-perceptions and how their communities and the larger world view the clients is useful in interpreting behaviors that white society might find inappropriate or perplexing. For example, what is called resistance, suspiciousness, or paranoia is often functional survival behavior for black clients.[18] The decades of overt and violent racism have caused black people to be sure of people's motive and to test relationships before developing trust in or becoming intimate with others. Asians, in contrast, survived by keeping a low profile. Their cultural values of respect for authority and politeness stimulate then to do the "right thing" to avoid losing face. Hence, they may smile and nod agreement even when they do not agree or understand.

Minority clients sometimes appear inappropriately angry or hostile. The anger they express may be an accumulation of repressed rage from numerous discriminatory experiences. Because it is often difficult for minority clients to distinguish between feelings generated by past and by present problems, it is important for the social worker to help them to do so and not be defensive or intimidated.

Although it is advantageous for the social worker and client to be of the same ethnic group, this is not necessarily the case for minority clients with AIDS in the initial phases of the relationship. Such clients sometimes fear that social workers from the same ethnic group would hold the prevailing attitudes of their community about AIDS and its associated high-risk behaviors. The minority therapists working with minority AIDS clients who were interviewed thought that the clients projected their judgments about themselves onto the therapists, so the initial sessions were spent in convincing the clients that the workers were actually supportive. Once the clients trusted the therapists, they found it reassuring to have someone of the same ethnicity who was helpful and might also be a positive role model.

Communication

White Americans place a greater emphasis than do minority clients on verbalizing feelings, open communication, and direct confrontation.[19] Black clients may emote while describing situations but not describe their actual feelings or thoughts; they think that their feelings are evident and consider their thoughts to be private. Asians are taught to control their feelings; thus, what appears to most non-Asians as a blunting of affect is really a reflection of control rather than the absence of feelings. Also, Asians believe that what is said is not as important as what is left unspoken. Hispanic men verbalize anger but rarely fear or anxiety.

For all minority clients, actions speak louder than words. Follow-up is important, as is the social worker's nonverbal behavior that is consistent with the feelings and opinions he or she has verbalized. Minority clients also value respect. To assume familiarity before being given permission is considered disrespectful. Furthermore, Asian and Hispanic clients often bring small gifts of food or other items to their worker rather than verbalize their appreciation. They perceive the refusal of a gift as a rejection of the gift giver; such as refusal, then, would alter, if not end, the relationship. For this reason, the social worker should never refuse refreshment during interviews with or home visits to minority AIDS clients.

Working with Families

Because families play such a large role in the lives of minority clients, working with the family or with client-family concerns is unavoidable. Whether or when to tell the family about the AIDS diagnosis and high-risk behaviors is a major issue that is complicated by the fact that many minority clients live with their parents and take care of them. Thus, they not only are afraid of being rejected but are concerned about who will provide for the parents if they are disowned or die. These clients generally have relied on their families for support all through their lives and may not have a reliable alternate support system, so they have more to lose than many other clients if they are rejected. It may take months for clients to decide how to disclose their situation to their families, and the decision often is influenced by the state of their health.

Because it is unacceptable for Asian and Hispanic families to reject an ill child, clients of these groups sometimes decide to tell their families of their diagnosis when they are so ill they can barely care for themselves. Although the families respond by providing care and shelter, they are not always able to provide emotional support. Therefore, when working with families, the social worker may find it helpful to minimize the stigma of AIDS and, in families in which role expectations are a sign of caring, focus on how well the client and his or her family have fulfilled the obligations they were able to fulfill and how they can continue to support each other as their roles require.

Whereas Asians tend to immigrate in families, many Hispanics do not. Those with families outside the United States usually do not tell their parents about their diagnosis unless their families already know they are gay. Many of their families cannot afford to visit them, so alternate support systems in the United States are essential. During the end stages of AIDS, most of these clients prefer to go home so they are with their families when they die. At this point, one's lifestyle and diagnosis are irrelevant, and there is no need to seek medical treatment or to fear rejection.

Several black clients said they would go to their families only as a last resort, and the author's experience has been that black families are not always as supportive as are Hispanic or Asian families. Black parents assume less responsibility for the actions of their adult children than do Asian and Hispanic parents, who would be judged overprotective by American standards. Adult black clients think they should be responsible for themselves and not have to depend on their parents. Moreover, blacks have been and are more stigmatized than are Asians and Hispanics and therefore have more reason to deny new problems that carry a stigma or to be defensive about them. The anger of the black community toward a black person with AIDS is more openly expressed and stems from the community's belief that the person and the diagnosis reinforce the unwanted perception that AIDS originated in black people, rather than that AIDS first appeared in Africa.

Other Concerns

Although churches are a strong source of support in minority communities, clients and their families do not feel comfortable seeking assistance from churches for AIDS-related concerns. They fear not only rejection by the congregation, but damnation for the person with AIDS. Churches in minority communities and the social service programs they run usually have not been available to minority clients with AIDS.

For monolingual clients, a translator may be necessary. With a subject as emotionally charged as AIDS and its associated high-risk behaviors, it is imperative to find a translator who can remain objective, supportive, and culturally sensitive. The translator must maintain strict confidentiality if he or she lives in the same ethnic community as the client. It is also important to evaluate the translator's knowledge and feelings about AIDS. Someone who is frightened or judgmental will not be able to translate accurately what the worker is saying. The use of a younger child as a translator is inappropriate; it would put an unfair burden on the child and make the parent feel that their authority was being undermined. The worker should discuss his or her expectations with the translator before they go to see the client together. A good translator can also be an excellent resource for learning more about a client's culture.

Whenever one works with clients from another culture, it is essential to evaluate their education, socioeconomic level, command of the English language, and level of acculturation. Family members adapt in different ways and to varying degrees—one may need to alter one's approach from client to client and from family member to family member. Differences in acculturation often lead to family conflicts, which can become more pronounced when a member is diagnosed as having AIDS. Clients who are more rooted in their ethnic community experience anxiety and a sense of loss over having to leave a secure environment to seek help in an unfamiliar one that may be unsupportive. The culturally sensitive social worker often becomes the cornerstone of an alternate support system for these clients.

Treatment modalities need to allow for cultural differences and cannot take a client out of the context of his ethnic background, community, and sexual lifestyle. A systems and problem-solving approach is effective, as is therapy that is directive, supportive, and short term. Group work can be effective if members are carefully screened for their level of acculturation, fluency in a common language, and willingness to participate. The group leader should be directive and focused and set a tone in which members do not feel overly pressured to reveal themselves or fearful of losing face. A more structured educational focus is useful at first because it provides a concrete service and an opportunity for group members to being to know each other.

Countertransference issues present a formidable challenge to practitioners. Working with minority clients with AIDS forces them to confront their feelings about AIDS, death and dying, ethnic minority groups, gay and bisexual people, substance abuse, family issues, unwed mothers, abortion, racism, and poverty. Because many clients are about the same age as the social workers, it is easy for the workers to overidentify or become overly involved with the clients, to burn out, or to forego the challenge and try to refer clients elsewhere. Workers also have to confront their tendency to view those who are different as inferior.

Conclusion

To preserve their cultural integrity and to ensure their survival, minority communities exert strong pressures on their members to conform to group norms. These pressures make the delivery of services to minority clients with AIDS a complex challenge that involves taking on taboos against gay and bisexual behaviors and the open discussion of sex, drugs, and AIDS. Agencies that are based in minority communities need to overcome their denial and fear of AIDS and to take more responsibility for developing culturally appropriate information about the disease and services to minority clients with AIDS. They have the cultural knowledge and community credibility to facilitate the creation of successful programs. Agencies in the larger community that deal with AIDS have the responsiblity to share their expertise and resources with the agencies in the minority communities and to make their services more culturally sensitive to minorities. Both types of agencies can learn from each other; working together is more cost effective and efficient and provides an opportunity to expand their perspectives and to overcome ethnic divisions and hostilities.

More funds should be allocated by the public and private sectors for education and services to minority communities in relation to AIDS with the stipulation that AIDS and minority-based agencies work together. A good relationship among the agencies can serve as a role model of trust and cooperation for community members who might then be encouraged to seek assistance.

Policies that seek to punish people with AIDS by denying them services or by restricting their civil rights will have devastating consequences for everyone. Such policies only increase hysteria, misinformation, and hostilities among different social groups. People who work in supportive environments have less of a tendency to engage in behaviors that are harmful to themselves and to others.

Working with minority clients with AIDS is a challenging opportunity for professional and personal growth. We social workers should not deny ourselves the experience because, in doing so, we only reflect the prejudices within ourselves and reinforce the fear of minority clients that we do not understand or care.

Notes and References

1. This information was gained by the author in a telephone call to the U.S. Bureau of the Census.

2. "AIDS Weekly Surveillance Report" (Atlanta, Ga.: Centers for Disease Control, June 30, 1986).

3. M. McGoldrick, J. Pearce, and J. Giordano, eds., *Ethnicity and Family Therapy* (New York: Guilford Press, 1982); F. Acosta, J. Yamamoto, and L. Evans, *Effective Psychotherapy for Low Income and Minority Patients* (New York: Plenum Press, 1982); and J. Oliver and L. Brown, eds., *Sociocultural and Service Issues in Working with Afro-American Clients* (New York: Rockefeller University Press, 1980).

4. "AIDS Weekly Surveillance Report."

5. These data were gathered by the author in a telephone call to the Centers for Disease Control.

6. S. P. Shon and D. Y. Ja, "Asian Families," in McGoldrick, Pearce, and Giordano, eds., *Ethnicity and Family Therapy,* pp. 211–212.

7. Ibid.

8. C. J. Falicon, "Mexican Families," in McGoldrick, Pearce, and Giordano, eds., p. 136.

9. Ibid.

10. D. Jones, "African-American Clients: Clinical Practice Issues," *Social Work,* 24 (March 1979), p. 113.

11. Ibid.

12. P. M. Hines and N. Boyd-Franklin, "Black Families," McGoldrick, Pearce, and Giordano, eds., *Ethnicity and Family Therapy,* p. 95.

13. "AIDS Weekly Surveillance Report."

14. Ibid.

15. Ibid.

16. Acosta, Yamamoto, and Evans, *Effective Psychotherapy for Low Income and Minority Patients,* p. 129.

17. *See* McGoldrick, Pearce, and Giordano, eds., *Ethnicity and Family Therapy*; Oliver and Brown, eds., *Sociocultural and Service Issues in Working with Afro-American Clients*; and ibid.

18. Jones, "Afro-American Clients," p. 115.

19. *For a more detailed discussion, see* Acosta, Yamamoto, and Evans, *Effective Psychotherapy for Low Income and Minority Patients.*

8

Social, Psychological, and Research Barriers to the Treatment of AIDS

Sr. Rosemary T. Moynihan and Grace H. Christ

Numerous practical, social, emotional, and attitudinal barriers must be overcome if AIDS is to be treated effectively and if the highest standards of medical and psychosocial care are to be achieved. Some of these barriers were identified in a study of the first 58 AIDS patients treated at Memorial Sloan-Kettering Cancer Center, New York City, between April 1981 and December 1982.[1] That study has been augmented by ongoing clinical assessments at the center and observations from practitioners in the New York City Social Work AIDS Network since 1983. These barriers include (1) cultural disynchrony with the health care staff; (2) reactions to disfigurement, deterioration, and death; (3) misperception of the modes of transmission of AIDS; (4) complicating social factors; and (5) limited support services. These barriers and the stresses caused by advances in research are discussed in this article, together with specialized interventions to address them.

Social and Psychological Barriers

Cultural Disynchrony

The diagnosis and treatment of AIDS requires continuous, intensely personal interactions between patients and the formal health care system.

Although health care institutions are a source of hope for cure and comfort for most ill people, this usually is not the case for AIDS patients because the health care staff often reject AIDS patients whose behavior and lifestyles are alien to the dominant culture of the staff. This disynchrony between AIDS patients and staff members causes many AIDS patients to be reluctant to or refuse to share personal information with physicians and hospitals because they are afraid that the loss of anonymity and confidentiality may lead to the loss of human rights—a loss that many AIDS patients have experienced and continue to experience.

Such disynchrony can be dismissed by individualizing the patients for staff—highlighting ways in which the patients' experiences and lifestyles are similar to those of the staff members, so the staff can more readily empathize with the patients. The staff must be willing to learn the language and culture of the gay and drug communities as they relate to their own; for example, lovers may be friends or permanent sexual partners, and drug use may be a mode of sharing. As the staff members being to see the needs and experiences that they and the patients have in common, their energy will be directed away from blame that distances them from the patients (for instance, "he brought this on himself" or "she destroyed her family with this destructive habit") and toward providing treatment and support. The following confrontation between the wife of an intravenous drug user with AIDS and a physician in an emergency room may serve as an example:

> The patient had become progressively demented and debilitated in the past six months, and his wife wanted him admitted to the hospital because of his mental confusion. The physician asked awkwardly, but with openness and some suspicion, "Why don't you people want to take your patients home?" "First of all," the wife replied, "What do you mean? Do you know what it's like to share a two-room apartment with two children and a dying, demented spouse with uncontrolled, contaminated diarrhea?" She went on to explain how she was fearful of AIDS for herself and her children, especially because of the uncontrolled diarrhea. The wife was angry and hurt at being so judged by the physician, who clearly spoke from a different life experience. The effect of the confrontation was to diminish immediately the barrier between them and to increase their mutual understanding.

Reactions to Disfigurement, Deterioration, and Death

The disfigurement; severe, often rapid, physical and mental deterioration; and high mortality rate of the young population of AIDS patients place extraordinary stress on health care staff, who become overwhelmed with sadness, a sense of helplessness, ineffectiveness, and hopelessness. The process of meeting young vital people and seeing them deteriorate physically and mentally (in Alzheimer's disease or Huntington's chorea) is more stressful than that of intervening at the terminal stage of an illness or with older dying patients with a lingering illness. In addition, the patients' closeness in age to that of the health care staff causes the staff to identify with the patients and consequently their fear of their own physical vulnerability.

These stresses must be recognized and addressed to prevent the staff from becoming emotionally overwhelmed and burned out because they often are important factors in the high turnover of staff who work with AIDS patients. Staff members are helped by learning about the underlying conceptual issues, by anticipating stress reactions, and by having the support of the administrators in developing stress-management skills.

Another important method of alleviating this kind of stress in the staff is to institute a cohesive, mutually supportive multidisciplinary team. The *Newsweek* article about the staff at Montefiore Hospital, New York City, contained a moving description of how the cohesiveness of the team served to buffer them against the overwhelming stresses of working with these patients and their families and friends.[2]

Misperceptions of the Modes of Transmission

Common misperceptions of the modes of transmission and the contagious potential of AIDS are another barrier to providing optimal services to AIDS patients. Although professionals are less likely now than they were early in the epidemic to refuse to care for AIDS patients, distancing and more indirect forms of resistance still occur. Repeated, clear, accurate information about contagion and transmission, given by knowledgeable medical authorities, mitigates the strong emotional responses that are responsible for misperceptions and distorted beliefs. Emphasizing that AIDS is a virus, rather than a lifestyle, an identity, or even an epidemic, is often helpful. Experience has demonstrated that the provision only of didactic information about the disease is of limited usefulness in dispelling distorted beliefs about the modes of transmission, even for physicians and nurses. Other means of helping staff deal with strong emotional reactions and stereotyped ideas need to be developed.

Complicating Factors

A number of social factors were identified early as significant barriers to obtaining optimal treatment and care.[3] First, many AIDS patients live alone and are socially isolated (with little or no access to community resources). Second, conflict or limited contact with biological families often creates additional challenges to coping at a time of physical and mental debilitation. Young adults with other serious illnesses often turn to their families of origin or a permanent lover as a major source of support. However, the families of AIDS patients often have rejected the patients' lifestyles or have not been aware of how the patients were living, and lovers frequently are afraid of contracting AIDS themselves. Therefore, the struggle to resolve these long-standing interpersonal issues at a time when medical treatment is so demanding requires great strength and energy. Furthermore, staff members frequently become involved in these struggles, which creates a level of intimacy between them and the patients that can hamper their maintenance of professional objectivity that is necessary when dealing with people in research or treatment.

Third, young people rarely have the financial resources or insurance to pay the exorbitant costs of treating AIDS, including the multiple medical crises, antibiotics and medications, hospital stays, and related expenses, such as transportation and at-home care. Their employment problems often reflect their limited work experience, the public's misconceptions of how the disease is transmitted, and prejudice. In addition, the erratic and often rapid onset of opportunistic infections can result in the intermittent availability for work. Thus, health care institutions must expand support services by working closely with community and city resources to assure continuing help for patients. In addition, the frequency of reports about the disease in the mass media often means that patients must continually hear or read news that confirms their poor prognosis and have little control over how and when they will confront the reality of their impending deaths—a control so important to terminally ill individuals.

Limited Support Services

Insufficient social-, home-care, and community-support services for patients, sexual partners, and families adds to the difficulty of providing effective treatment to AIDS patients. In New York City, which has the largest population of AIDS patients in the country, few chronic and terminal care beds or supervised living situations are willing to accept these patients.[4] Most patients receive professional care at home, alone or with their families, from the Visiting Nurse Service, Medicaid and Medicare services, or from some proprietary nursing agencies. The demands on families and friends are enormous, and there are few respite services or resources for them. Furthermore, the lack of aftercare or discharge care makes hospitals more hesitant and less able to take on new cases that ultimately will drain their resources and not be reimbursed.

Emerging Research-related Issues

Treatment for the Underlying Immunodeficiency

Despite the expansion of medical research on AIDS and the development of many more potential treatment interventions, there is still no cure for AIDS. Furthermore, all treatments for the underlying immunodeficiency are still being conducted under research conditions using a double-bind strategy with a placebo, and they are Phase I status research; that is, the goal is to demonstrate some effect on the disease process in humans. In this high-tech age, in which answers to most problems seem to be possible and to be gained rapidly, patients and those at risk of contracting AIDS often attribute the lack of effective treatment to a lack of intense effort or a disinterest in saving their lives because of their minority social status. Their anger and hopelessness can be mitigated if they are allowed to exercise some denial or at times adaptive avoidance and if their physicians continuously reassure them of their interest and concern.

Moreover, that the treatments address symptoms, related infections, fungi, and cancers, rather than the immunodeficiency, often confuses patients about the meaning of treatment and the nature of the illness. The patients may try to cope with this reality and confusion by focusing their hope on the treatment of specific complications, such as pneumocystis carinii pneumonia. Then, when confronted with other medical crises that heighten their awareness of the underlying immunodeficiency, they feel let down and betrayed. To defend themselves against this constant threat to their lives, many patients go from one institution to another trying different, sometimes holistic, treatments—often the latest ones hyped by the media. Unfortunately, this search for alternative remedies often complicates and invalidates the studies that are attempting to find a cure. Consequently, the admissions criteria of most research projects are becoming more stringent. The reliance on alternative treatments has a more immediate detrimental effect on patients as well; it can delay the effective treatment of reversible infections or medical complications and hence result in premature death.

Problems of Human Experimentation

Some unique problems arise in the course of the research of AIDS. First, especially on the East Coast and West Coast, people with AIDS and those at a high risk of contracting it are generally in minority social groups. After decades of experience, these groups have learned to fear that human experiments do not always regard the well-being of their subjects. In addition, they are afraid that the information they disclose to the researchers will be given to governmental and private groups and that the disclosure of this confidential information will lead to the loss of their rights or to their incarceration. This fear is making potential and actual participants in research projects increasingly hesitant to divulge personal information that is necessary for conducting the research, especially that relate to sexual practices, sexual partners, transmission patterns, and patterns of drug traffic. This fear also hampers the researchers' efforts to trace and educate those who are at risk of contracting AIDS because of their contact with the patients.

Second, many AIDS patients find it difficult to comply with the stringent requirements of the research treatment. For both the young gay and bisexual men and the intravenous drug users, who are constantly confronted with multiple medical crises, this discipline demands great ego strength, adaptive denial, motivation, and trust. However, the intravenous drug users bear an additional burden as well: the demands of their addiction and its treatment. In the past few years, more has been learned about people with minority lifestyles and addictions. Thus, although many patients who are self-destructive can be motivated by their concern for hurting others, it has been found that the timing and goals of education should be focused on such reasonable steps as the use of clean needles rather than stopping the use of drugs, or anticipating the regression related to the progression of the disease and the painful side effects of treatment.

Third, the end of research treatment or protocols often means the loss of structured emotional support and of the sense that the disease is being controlled. Although they are relieved by the lack of symptoms, patients must now face the reality that little more can be done other than tenuous research treatments and the management of future symptoms. To deal with the trauma brought about by the end of treatment, many patients maintain close contact with health care and mental health staff for reassurance that they will receive help when they again become sick or are dying.

Side Effects

The treatments themselves create some expected and unexpected problems. For example, chemotherapy causes such side effects as nausea, vomiting, mouth sores, and the loss of hair and appetite. Radiation therapy requires multiple, often lengthy, visits to the hospital and results in exhaustion, nausea, and burns; furthermore, patients are frustrated to learn that radiation affects only the symptoms of local diseases, such as the lesions on the face, eyes, mouth, esophagus, or feet of Kaposi's sarcoma.

Less familiar and, at times, more complicated problems occur with Phase I, Phase II, or less traditional treatments. The media hype of interferon as a "wonder drug" was chastened by the unexpected organically caused depression that accompanied the administration of this substance, and it took quite a while to identify this effect of the treatment. Intervention with appropriate psychotropic drugs could only be determined after other variables were examined that could have caused reactive depression. The initial treatment with interferon required daily injections at the hospital for several months, which resulted in constant flulike symptoms. Such a regimen eliminated the possibility of adaptive avoidance because patients were confronted daily with their symptoms and they were confused about what was causing their symptoms: the disease or its treatment. Bone marrow transplantation—another type of treatment—requires the total physical isolation of patients. It is especially difficult for AIDS patients because it exacerbates the social isolation they have been experiencing because of AIDS and that they have experienced because of their sexual identity or lifestyle.

Ambiguous Health Status

The ambiguity in the diagnosis of the disease also creates confusion and is stressful to those affected. Patients with lymphadenopathy or ARC demonstrate even higher levels of anxiety and depression than do patients with a definite diagnosis of AIDS because of the added uncertainty but increased possibility of contracting AIDS.[5] Tests of the blood of potential blood donors for signs of the HIV or HTLV-III virus have created another group of anxious and confused individuals. Because of the need to protect the blood supply, this gross screen was developed to eliminate any indications of the disease. Despite its nondiagnostic status, this type of blood test is being used as a screen. However, individuals who test positive were told they could be false positives, could be carriers of the disease, or could never have it. Individuals could also have the disease and not be identified by the test. However, with use, scientists have become more confident of the accuracy of the test, and it seems more likely that those who have the antibody also have the virus. Furthermore, even people with a diagnosis of AIDS, especially those whose initial illness is Kaposi's sarcoma, may have few or no other symptoms to indicate their illness and hence may wonder whether they are still sick if they do not have symptoms. The vulnerability of an underlying immune status is difficult to conceptualize and integrate, especially for people so young.

Under such uncertain conditions, social and interpersonal contacts and relationships are complicated. Individuals ask questions such as these: Can I have traditional sexual contact? Should I tell potential sexual partners about my condition, however uncertain it may be? Should I become pregnant? What are the risks to my unborn child? How should I handle a medical examination for a new job? These situations have created a need for new counseling strategies to help people cope with the anxiety and stress caused by the ambiguity of their social, emotional, and possibly financial, employment, and political states, which may continue throughout the estimated incubation period of four or more years.

Longer Survival Time

Medical research has made rapid progress against the virus despite what seems to be an interminable period of human devastation. The virus has been identified, isolated, and grown and the information base has vastly increased. Moreover, progress in the refinement of antibiotics and chemotherapeutic and antifungal agents has increased the survival time of AIDS patients. However, the promise of longer survival is compromised by debilitating mental conditions that become increasingly severe and the burden of further higher medical costs.

One of the most difficult problems for patients, caregivers, and staff stemming from the longer survival time is the advancing neurological impairment. In the earliest phases, abnormalities, including difficulty in remembering telephone numbers, names, or appointments and in keeping track of communications, may be mild and can be misconstrued as general psychological reactions to illness, general malaise, or reactive depression. Such symptoms as frustration and bewilderment in trying to follow a sequential task may appear even before a specific diagnosis. Gradually, the patients' verbal and motor responses become slower and less sponteneous. In the advanced states of AIDS, the most frequent symptoms are apathy, withdrawal, and a loss of interest; less frequent complications are organic psychosis, agitation, inappropriate behavior, and hallucinations.

Apathy and withdrawal usually oscillate with the final severe cognitive impairment and psychomotor slowing.[6] Because the patients are young, it is harder for caretakers and health care personnel to accept these symptoms of dementia, which usually are seen in the elderly, middle-aged patients with Alzheimer's disease, or patients with Huntington's chorea. The concomitant personality changes often confuse and distance caretakers and make the provision of home health care more difficult to deliver.

Thus, the longer survival of patients and the hope it evokes are compromised by the destruction of the quality of the patient's life. New resources need to be developed to deal with the complications created by advances in research. As important is the development of counseling techniques that are effective in helping those who are slowly being denied their personalities as well as their lives and the complex emotional needs of their survivors.

Finally, the enormous financial costs of health care to people with AIDS is of concern not only to patients and institutions but to the whole society. Most gay men with AIDS are young and gainfully employed, but they use up their insurance quickly. They are unfamiliar with city, state, and federal agencies that provide financial assistance and require advocacy and emotional support to deal with them. Furthermore, insurance companies use various excuses to deny the claims of AIDS patients such as a preexisting illness or an unclear diagnosis. Although many drug users are on Medicaid, Medicaid does not cover the necessary level of home care for them. Counseling needs abound for parents and significant others, many of whom require psychiatric treatment and medication; however, again, these costs are reimbursed at low levels. Hospital, mental health, and medical financial resources are inadequate to meet these ongoing and increasing needs.

Intervention

Prevention

Although we social workers must continue to direct considerable efforts toward using our traditional mental health skills on behalf of this fatally ill young population, we must develop new means of intervention to deal with the unique problems of AIDS patients. One such avenue is primary prevention. Rarely has primary prevention been so clear a means of containing a disease as it is with AIDS. Social workers have always been active in secondary and tertiary prevention to minimize the impact of a disease and to maximize the potential and quality of life of the ill person; however, primary prevention presents new challenges.

What are these preventive tasks and how can we help? Many of the high-risk behaviors that require modificiation (including sexual behavior and drug use) are central to the identities and lifestyles of the two main groups of AIDS patients—gay men and intravenous drug users. In addition, these necessary behavioral changes often involve interactions with others so that individuals need help to manage their relationships as well as to change their personal habits.

Social workers are uniquely sensitized and trained to help individuals with both these tasks, but new and creative interventions must be developed to address the needs of these specific populations. For example, we must learn ways to identify individuals who are at risk and help them deal with their high-risk behaviors. However, this task can evoke strong feelings of countertransference that must be acknowledged. The identification of gay or bisexual men or those who have had a bisexual experience and of those who have used intravenous drugs and the evaluation of such issues as how sexual partners are chosen challenge professional and personal values. Yet, because of these individuals' fear of rejection, some of this information may be brought out unless it is actively sought—but it must be sought in a climate of the acceptance of these individuals' lifestyles and behaviors.

Psychosocial research is beginning to provide us with some information that can be integrated into our interventive strategies so that preventive interventions are grounded in both clinical insight and research findings. For example, it has been found that education has been helpful in promoting some changes in behavior, but only to a limited extent.[7] It also has been found that asymptomatic gay men changed their sexual practices to the extent that these changes did not significantly interfere with their lifestyles and did not cause them major psychological and social discomfort.[8] Clearly, if additional changes are required, other forms of support for behavioral modifications are necessary in addition to the giving of information.

An important issue to be considered in preventive intervention is the role of "denial"—a concept that has been much debated in the treatment of cancer. It generally is agreed that the use of denial when confronting an uncontrollable situation is often adaptive. However, because AIDS is preventable, risk groups must be continuously aware of the dangers involved in specific behaviors.

Most mental health interventions are aimed at reducing anxiety, but Siegel's research with healthy gay men showed that individuals who engaged in the most risk-taking behaviors had the lowest anxiety and the most inaccurate perception of their risk and that those who confronted the threat of AIDS and were more likely to initiate and maintain safe sexual practices had higher levels of anxiety.[9] Thus, anxiety can be viewed as an important motivating force for practicing safe sex and protecting one's health. It may promote vigilance and the maintenance of behavioral patterns that lower the risk of contracting AIDS.

Moderate, fear-inducing health-education strategies are probably necessary to motivate gay and bisexual men to limit themselves to safer practices. However, the psychological distress caused by these strategies is high. We need to develop ways for gay and bisexual men to accomplish the difficult dual tasks of maintaining a level of anxiety sufficient to motivate safe sex and managing anxiety and maintaining psychological equilibrium. A second factor associated with the reduction of risk behaviors in Siegel's study was the presence of good social skills.[10] Those who could openly negotiate changes with others and relate on many different levels were better able to give up dangerous sexual practices and find alternative means of gratification. These concepts guide the management of nontraditional ongoing support groups that provide accurate information on AIDS, teach social skills, help individuals maximize their personal resources as a means not only of motivating behavioral change but of moderating anxiety caused by heightened awareness of the consequences of behavior, reducing social isolation, and developing new social networks.

Another factor that is consistently associated with the reduction of risk behaviors is the support of reference group norms. Clearly, with interactive behaviors, a group's sanction of such basic changes is vital. Interventions that are aimed at enhancing a group's support of risk-reduction behaviors are likely to help individuals in the group who may be better able to make changes if they can still feel accepted and valued by their peers. For instance, Gay Men's Health Crisis in New York City uses the following slogan: "Condoms are bringing men back together again"; the center uses safety pins to symbolize its sanction of safer sex and emphasizes and affirms the value of ongoing relationships. Gay sex films and cable television shows are now often explicit about high-risk behaviors and suggest substitute behaviors. One television show ended by saying: "Hey, if you don't want to change, then die!" Although such a saying is clearly a negative sanction, the show also emphasized the erotic quality of alternative sexual behaviors and group acceptance of these new behaviors.

Preventive interventions also need to include a thorough understanding of the various cultures involved so that individuals can be helped to adapt creatively to the realities of the disease by finding options that are acceptable to them and to their reference group. The following case is an example:

> Mrs. B—a young black women who was an ex-drug addict—gave birth to a baby who was diagnosed as having AIDS. Her bout with drugs occurred five years earlier during a period of severe adolescent turmoil. Since then, she obtained a nursing degree and married a sensitive and caring man whose maturity seemed much beyond his 23 years. When this young woman was found to be HIV positive, her husband was told

not to have sex with her; he responded by saying that he did not want to be a "monk." Mrs. B then went through a period of severe depression and acting out, desperately wanting to remain with her husband but fearing she would transmit the disease to him. An evaluation of the actual risk of her transmitting the disease led to suggestions that the couple use condoms and change of some of their specific sexual behaviors.

Although the relationship was stabilized, these changes and the implicit threat continued to impose stress on their marriage. However, this more gradual approach within the context of the couples' milieu and culture offered at least some hope of their maintaining a supportive relationship.

Complicating Medical and Social Factors

In addition to incorporating knowledge about AIDS, it is vital that clinical interventions integrate knowledge about a host of complicating medical and social factors. Thus, social workers who work with AIDS patients must not only become informed about the knowledge base of other social work specializations but must develop networks and act as liaisons with new professional and political groups and individuals. Although these activities may not be new to social workers, who have always dealt with the social complexity of different cultures and multiproblem situations, they are especially challenging to and often overlooked by those who work with AIDS patients.

One such complicating factor involved hemophiliacs. The majority of hemophiliacs in the United States are antibody positive for the virus because of their essential infusions with Factor VIII. After already having adapted to one life-threatening disease, they must learn to live with the ongoing uncertainty about contracting AIDS. Worry about the health of sexual partners and anger over the unfairness of their exposure that causes them to be confronted with new social prejudice adds to the stress of an already tenuous adjustment to a hereditary blood disorder.

The medical treatment for AIDS of intravenous drug users and gay men is complicated by similar and no-so-similar problems. Both groups are concerned about sexual relations. Intravenous drug users, in addition, worry about endangering any children they might bear, despite the social stereotype of them as rejecting personal and social responsibilities. Furthermore, current or previous drug addiction can cause complex medical treatment problems because medications for pain, psychotropic drugs, and some anti-emetic drugs have cross tolerance with addictive substances, and it is difficult to continue to maintain addicts on methadone while medicating them for AIDS. The effective treatment of AIDS demands a high level of compliance for a limited outcome, which individuals who already have demonstrated problems with controlling the gratification of impulses and with tolerating emotional and physical frustration find it difficult to do.

The gay community has developed a culture, network, and language that bonds its members as protection against an often-hostile majority culture. The treatment of AIDS requires sharing intimate and personal information with health care professionals who are often heterosexual. Unconscious prejudice and personal differences can contribute to the emotional distance of staff members when patients are already struggling with guilt, shame, and fear related to the disease and its implications.

Minority groups, especially minority women, are at risk of contracting AIDS because the majority of intravenous drug users in such large cities as New York, Jersey City, Los Angeles, and Miami are minority men. Despite increased efforts to educate minority women about safer sexual practices, these women have been difficult to reach. Their fear of the loss of income, emotional support, being left alone, and physical abuse and their perceptions of the limited options open to them undermine their development of more self-protective behaviors.

Professionals in specialized areas of medicine and mental health, treatment groups, institutions, drug rehabilitation centers, and community services must continue to develop effective strategies for sharing information and planning systems of education and support. Without such systems, we may unwittingly undermine drug treatment efforts, create a fragmented treatment process that overwhelms patients who are suffering from dementia, or weaken the effectivenss of existing services. Co-coverage of patients often requires breaking through traditional professional barriers; thus, for example, drug rehabilitation counselors or specialized medical personnel must be more than visitors in the health or mental health setting.

Development of Resources

Although direct clinical interventions by professionals are vital, they are one aspect of the multidimensional approach necessary to meet the complex needs previously discussed. Therefore, some different strategies must be considered. For example, traditional practitioners must join in developing and affirming new social networks, such as pride programs sponsored by the gay and lesbian communities, ex-addict-to-addict programs like ADAPT, and patient/family self-help groups to compensate for inadequate or nonexistent resources. These networks can provide practical help in addition to emotional support and, in some situations, can function as surrogate families. For instance, the mother of a now-dead 23-year-old addict with AIDS started a parents self-help group for moral support of and referrals from the staff at Memorial Sloan-Kettering Cancer Center. Because of her nonthreatening approach and her familiarity with their situation, she succeeded (where professionals had failed) in drawing out frightened, isolated parents.

In any treatment setting, it is necessary for all AIDS patients to be helped to apply soon after their diagnosis for financial entitlements, especially for disabilty insurance under Social Security, Supplemental Security Income, and Medicaid. Although this type of help may seem to be a misuse of treatment time it is not; because of the immunodeficiency, the course of the disease is erratic, and the onset of overwhelming opportunistic infections often is rapid. The early application for financial assistance can be presented to patients as an insurance to fall back on because such applications usually are a frightening confirmation of their disease to newly diagnosed or asymptomatic patients. This kind of conceptual framework allows for acceptance of the need for planning while supporting adaptive denial at earlier stages. The case of Andrew may serve as an example:

> Andrew was without symptoms for two years. He decided to depend on Blue Cross/Blue Shield from his job as a college professor, which seemed adequate for the current state of his disease. His therapist supported this avoidance as adaptive without helping him to address the necessary tasks and was unprepared when Andrew experienced a progressive dementia over a two-week period that necessitated round-the-clock care.

This kind of situation is less likely to occur if private therapists, mental health agencies, and hospital staff help patients obtain basic financial entitlements and practical assistance as part of ongoing counseling, rather than divide care into traditional counseling and concrete services.

Furthermore, the recent shift of medical treatment and care to the home confronts patients and staff alike with new, at times, overwhelming, deficits in resources. Treatments that formerly were given in the hospital, such as antibiotics administered intravenously, antifungal agents, chemotherapy, and nutrition, are now being delivered at home, where resources often are inadequate. Highly technical forms of treatment can be frightening to manage and require close communication with professional health care staff. Although mental health practitioners can do little about this problem, they can help family members deal with their emotional needs surrounding these tasks if they are aware of this situation.

In addition, AIDS patients whose survival has been prolonged but who are mentally and physically deteriorated require continuous supervision or chronic care. In most cities, housing and chronic care facilities are either not available or inadequate for AIDS patients. Therefore, many patients are forced to stay in isolated hospital rooms when supervised care would be sufficient and would provide a better quality of life. A continuum of care, including acute care, supervised living, and chronic care facilities; nursing homes; hospices are required in every community to meet the needs of this population of patients.

Conclusion

As this article has shown, social workers are challenged to develop interventions that will help overcome the social and psychological barriers to the optimal treatment and care of AIDS patients. In addition, we must help to mitigate the impact of the stresses created by necessary advances in research.

All social workers—not only those who specialize in the treatment of AIDS patients—will be affected by the epidemic and need to be informed of the disease and its modes of transmission, as well as its psychosocial impact on patients, their families and friends, and society in general because they will come into contact with the families and friends of AIDS patients, individuals with a positive antibody test, members of at-risk groups, and the worried well. The complex practical, social, psychological, and ethical issues confronting these individuals and health professionals challenge the depth and breadth of our knowledge, skills, and commitment to human concerns, as does the need to fulfill the public health goal of primary prevention. Social workers are in a unique position to support the development of comprehensive systems of care for AIDS patients, to humanize medical research, to bridge the gap between science and the individual experience, and to assist in preventing the spread of this disease because of their experience with and skills in addressing multiple systems and their impact on the individual.

Notes and References

1. G. H. Christ and L. S. Wiener, "Psychosocial Issues in AIDS," in V. T. DeVita, S. Hellman, and S. A. Rosenberg, eds., *AIDS: Etiology, Diagnosis, Treatment and Prevention* (Philadelphia: J.B. Lippincott Co., 1985), pp. 275–297.

2. P. Goldman and L. Beachy, "One Against the Plague," *Newsweek,* July 21, 1986, pp. 38–50.

3. G. H. Christ, L. S. Wiener, and R. T. Moynihan, "Psychosocial Issues in AIDS," *Psychiatric Annals,* 16 (March 1986), pp. 173–179.

4. H. M. Ginzburg and M. G. MacDonald, "The Epidemiology of Human T-Cell Lymphotropic Virus, Type III (HTLV-III Disease)," *Psychiatric Annals,* 16 (March 1986), pp. 153–157.

5. J. C. Holland and S. Tross, "The Psychosocial and Neuropsychiatric Sequelae of the Acquired Immunodeficiency Syndrome and Related Disorders," *Annals of Internal Medicine,* 103 (November 1985), pp. 760–764.

6. B. Navia and R. W. Price, "Dementia Complicating AIDS," *Psychiatric Annals,* 16 (March 1986), pp. 158–166.

7. L. J. Bauman and K. Siegel, "Misperception Among Gay Men of the Risk for AIDS Associated with Their Sexual Behavior," *Journal of Applied Social Psychology,* in press.

8. L. McKusick et al., "AIDS and Sexual Behavior reported by Gay Men in San Francisco," *American Journal of Public Health,* 15 (May 1985),

pp. 493–496; and K. Siegel and L. J. Bauman, "Sexual Practices of Gay and Bisexual Men in New York City," paper at a meeting of the American Sociological Association, New York, New York, August 1986.

9. K. Siegel, "AIDS: The Social Dimension," *Psychiatric Annals,* 16 (March 1986), pp. 168–172.

10. Ibid.

Contributors

Robert J. Battjes, DSW, Associate Director of Planning, Division of Clinical Research, National Institute on Drug Abuse, U.S. Public Health Service, Rockville, Maryland

Esther Chachkes, MSW, Assistant Director, Department of Social Work, Montefiore Hospital, Medical Center–Moses Division, Bronx, New York

Grace H. Christ, MSW, Director, Department of Social Work, Memorial Sloan–Kettering Cancer Center, New York, New York

Manuel Fimbres, MSW, Professor, San José State University, Graduate School of Social Work, San José, California

Sally Jue, MSW, Associate Director of Client Services for the AIDS Project of Los Angeles, West Hollywood, California

Carl G. Leukefeld, DSW, Chief Health Services Officer and Deputy Director, Division of Clinical Research, National Institute on Drug Abuse, U.S. Public Health Service, Rockville, Maryland

Judy Macks, MSW, Director of Mental Health Training, AIDS Health Project, San Francisco, California

Sr. Rosemary T. Moynihan, MSW, Assistant Director, Department of Social Work, Memorial Sloan–Kettering Cancer Center, New York, New York

Deborah A. Newmark, Clinical Social Worker, Social Work Department, National Institutes of Health, Bethesda, Maryland

Caitlin C. Ryan, MSW, President, Healthsource, Inc., Washington, D.C.

Martin Schwartz, Ed.D., Professor of Social Work, Virginia Commonwealth University, Richmond, Virginia

Edward H. Taylor, Ph.D., Clinical and Research Social Worker, National Institute of Mental Health, Neuropsychiatric Branch, Saint Elizabeths Hospital, Washington, D.C.

Positions are those held at the time of the conference.